Common Medical Conditions

A Guide for the Dental Team

Stephen C. Bain
Swansea University

John Hamburger
University of Birmingham

Crispian Scully
University College London

⊛WILEY-BLACKWELL
A John Wiley & Sons, Ltd., Publication

Blackwell Publishing was acquired by John Wiley & Sons in February 2007. Blackwell's publishing programme has been merged with Wiley's global Scientific, Technical, and Medical business to form Wiley-Blackwell.

Registered office
John Wiley & Sons Ltd, The Atrium, Southern Gate, Chichester, West Sussex, PO19 8SQ, United Kingdom

Editorial offices
9600 Garsington Road, Oxford, OX4 2DQ, United Kingdom
2121 State Avenue, Ames, Iowa 50014-8300, USA

For details of our global editorial offices, for customer services and for information about how to apply for permission to reuse the copyright material in this book please see our website at www.wiley.com/wiley-blackwell.

Library of Congress Cataloging-in-Publication Data
Bain, Steve, MA.
    Common medical conditions : a guide for the dental team / S. Bain, J. Hamburger, C. Scully.
        p. ; cm.
    Includes bibliographical references and index.
    ISBN 978-1-4051-8593-6 (hardback : alk. paper)   1. Oral manifestations of general diseases.
2. Internal medicine. 3. Dentists. I. Hamburger, John. II. Scully, Crispian. III. Title.
    [DNLM: 1. Oral Manifestations. 2. Dental Care. WU 290 B162c 2010]
    RK305.B35 2010
    616–dc22

                                                                                        2009033617

A catalogue record for this book is available from the British Library.

Set in 10/12 pt Sabon by SNP Best-set Typesetter Ltd., Hong Kong
Printed in Singapore

1 2010

Contents

Preface

This book, written by clinicians from different backgrounds, specialising in medicine and/or oral medicine, summarises the medical problems that are considered to be most common and/or important in the developed countries. The concept arose from two series of papers written by the authors for Dental Update.

The clinical presentation, physical signs, diagnosis, management and oral health care relevance of 50 of the mainly acquired and chronic conditions are described. The text is presented in 10 chapters, illustrated with examples of clinical signs predominantly involving those areas of the body that are most readily accessible and easily visible to dental health care professionals – mainly the face, neck and limbs.

This book should be of value to undergraduate and postgraduate dental professionals, and junior hospital dental staff and additionally as a succinct and accessible reference text for the general dental practitioner and team.

Stephen C. Bain
John Hamburger
Crispian Scully

1

Cardiovascular conditions

Atheroma

Atheroma (atherosclerosis) is characterised by the accumulation of cholesterol and lipids in the arterial intimal surface. Atheroma has a patchy distribution and, depending on the site and extent of disease, can give rise to a variety of clinical presentations (Table 1.1). A platelet–fibrin thrombus (clot) may form, break up and travel in the bloodstream (thrombo-embolism) with potentially life-threatening consequences. Alternatively, atheromatous plaques may rupture and 'heal' spontaneously.

Table 1.1   Common sites of atheroma and clinical presentation

Artery site	Clinical presentation
Cerebral	Cerebrovascular accident – stroke
	Transient ischaemic attacks (TIAs)
Coronary	Coronary artery disease – chest pain (angina pectoris)
	Arrhythmias
	Myocardial infarction
Peripheral	Intermittent claudication
	Resting leg pain
	Infarction leading to gangrene

Coronary artery disease

Coronary artery disease (CAD) is caused by atheroma. It is the leading cause of death in the UK and results from a combination of genetic and lifestyle factors. Irreversible (fixed) risk factors include:

- Increasing age
- Gender: men are at greater risk than premenopausal women
- Family history of CAD.

Potentially reversible (modifiable) risk factors for CAD include:

- Cigarette smoking
- High blood cholesterol level: low density lipoproteins (LDL) are associated with a high risk of CAD, whilst high density lipoproteins (HDL) appear to be anti-atherogenic

- Hypertension
- Diabetes mellitus
- Obesity and lack of exercise.

Clinical features

The clinical presentation of CAD is reflective of the degree and duration of impaired coronary blood flow. Features include dizziness, shortness of breath, decreased exercise tolerance, chest pain (angina pectoris) and sometimes sudden death due to a catastrophic myocardial infarction (irreversible damage to cardiac muscle). Xanthelasmata may signify hyperlipidaemia. A chronically reduced blood supply to the myocardium progressively damages the heart muscle and may lead to cardiac arrhythmias and cardiac failure.

Clinical signs

Distended neck veins (Figure 1.1) due to increased jugular venous pressure (JVP), are a classic sign of right-sided cardiac failure, although it may also be seen in hypervolaemic states, superior vena cava obstruction and cardiac tamponade. The causes of cardiac failure may also include cardiac valvular disease

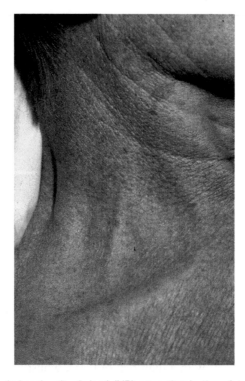

Figure 1.1   Distended neck veins (raised JVP) are a classic sign of right-sided cardiac failure

and chronic obstructive pulmonary disease. Pitting oedema may be demonstrated by applying firm digital pressure over the lower legs or ankles.

Hyperlipidaemia may predispose to CAD [sometimes premature]. The combination of corneal arcus with xanthelasma (Figure 1.2) should suggest the possibility of hyperlipidaemia. This is especially the case in young people where autosomal dominant familial hypercholesterolaemia may be the underlying cause. Other causes of xanthelasma (but not corneal arcus) include hypothyroidism and primary biliary cirrhosis.

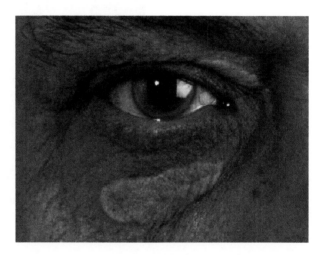

Figure 1.2 Hyperlipidaemia is suggested by the combination of corneal arcus with xanthelasma

It is thought that if an individual has diagonal creases (Figure 1.3) on both ear lobes, there may be some benefit in undergoing screening to exclude the possibility of cardiovascular disease. The actual cause of earlobe creasing is unknown but it is possible that chronic circulatory problems allow the vascular bed in the earlobe to collapse and the telltale earlobe crease to appear. In one study the presence of a unilateral earlobe crease was associated with a 33% increase in the risk of a myocardial infarct; the risk increased to 77% when the earlobe crease appeared bilaterally.

Vertex baldness also appears to be a valid marker for an increased risk of cardiovascular disease, particularly when clustered with other factors such as hypertension or hypercholesterolaemia. Other factors include being short and having an 'apple-shaped' physique.

The American Academy of Periodontology recently showed that people with periodontal disease are 200–300% more likely to experience a heart attack than those with healthy periodontium, making periodontal disease a possible risk for cardiovascular disease.

Atheroma, trauma, orbital apex disease, cavernous sinus disease, aneurysm of the posterior communicating artery, raised intracranial pressure and diabetes (often a partial palsy) are all possible causes of a third nerve (oculomotor) palsy

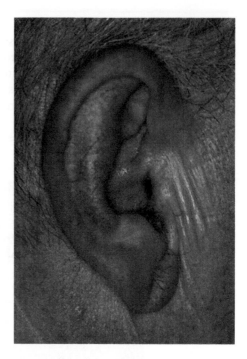

Figure 1.3   Creases in the earlobe may indicate cardiovascular disease

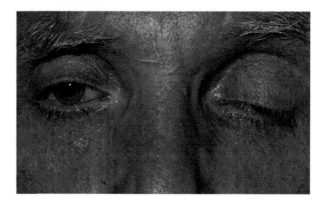

Figure 1.4   A left-sided third cranial nerve palsy

(Figure 1.4). The third nerve supplies all of the muscles of the orbit apart from the superior oblique (IV cranial nerve) and the lateral rectus (VI). Unopposed action of these muscles leads to the eye pointing 'down and out'. It is also the muscle that raises the eyelid (levator palpebrae), the ciliary muscle and constrictor of the pupil, hence there is a complete ptosis (drooping of the eyelid) and dilatation of the pupil. The left eye would be looking inferolaterally ('down and out') giving a divergent squint and the pupil would be dilated (complete paralysis) or normal ('partial third nerve palsy').

Diagnosis

- Clinical history.
- Electrocardiogram (ECG): the resting ECG may be normal and so an exercise ECG is also indicated.
- Myocardial perfusion scans (thallium-201) show ischaemic areas as 'cold spots' during exercise.
- Coronary angiography assesses the coronary artery anatomy and patency.

Management

Emphasis should be on lifestyle changes with the primary aim to prevent, or reduce progression of, coronary atheroma. These include:

- Dietary modification: reduction of cholesterol and saturated fat intake
- Regular exercise
- Weight loss
- Smoking cessation.

Pharmacological measures for the management of CAD include:

- Anti-platelet drugs (aspirin or clopidogrel)
- Anti-hypertensive treatment with beta-blockers (atenolol), diuretics (furosemide) and angiotensin converting enzyme (ACE) inhibitors (enalapril)
- Cholesterol lowering drugs such as statins (simvastatin)
- Good control of blood glucose levels if diabetic.

When CAD is extensive and an individual's symptoms are worsening despite general measures and optimal medical management, cardiac revascularisation techniques that should be considered include:

- Coronary angioplasty: stents may be placed percutaneously (percutaneous coronary intervention [PCI]), to re-establish coronary blood flow and improve myocardial perfusion
- Coronary artery bypass grafts (CABGs) to bridge severe obstructions in the coronary blood vessels.

Angina pectoris

Angina pectoris is the name given to episodes of chest pain caused by myocardial ischaemia secondary to CAD. Angina affects around 1% of the adult population and its prevalence rises with increasing age. The severity and prognosis of angina depends upon the degree of coronary artery narrowing and has a varied clinical presentation. The average annual mortality rate in the UK is about 4% per year.

Clinical features

Angina is often unmistakable because the pain is precipitated by physical exertion, particularly in cold weather, and is relieved by rest. Affected individuals

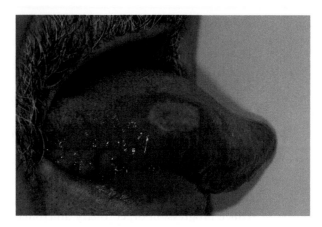

Figure 1.5   Severe oral ulceration caused by nicorandil

may describe a sense of tightness, heaviness, compression or constriction of the chest, sometimes radiating to the left arm or jaw. Emotion (anger or anxiety) and stress (fear or pain) can induce angina by leading to the release of catecholamines (epinephrine [adrenaline] and norepinephrine [noradrenaline]) from the adrenal cortex. These hormones result in an increased heart rate (tachycardia), a raised blood pressure (reactive hypertension), and vasoconstriction of the coronary circulation. Consequently an increased cardiac workload is accompanied by a paradoxical drop in blood flow and myocardial ischaemia occurs – resulting in angina.

Variants of angina include:

- Stable angina: pain only on exertion and relieved in a few minutes by rest and sublingual glyceryl trinitrate (GTN)
- Decubitus angina: pain on lying down
- Vasospastic (variant or Prinzmetal) angina: caused by coronary artery spasm
- Acute coronary syndrome (unstable angina): angina at rest or of sudden onset with a rapid increase in severity. This is due to a transient subtotal obstruction of a coronary vessel and is a medical emergency
- Cardiac syndrome X: clinical features of angina but normal coronary arteries on angiogram. It is thought to be due to a functional abnormality of the coronary microcirculation.

Clinical signs

Some drugs such as nicorandil used in the management of unstable angina, can produce severe oral ulceration (Figure 1.5).

Diagnosis

The diagnosis of angina is primarily a clinical one. Physical examination and investigations may be normal. The individual's risk factors for CAD should be carefully assessed. Investigations may include:

- Resting electrocardiogram (ECG): during pain there may be ST segment depression with a flat or inverted T-wave. The ECG is usually normal between episodes of angina
- Exercise ECG testing: positive in approximately 75% of people with severe CAD
- Myocardial perfusion scans (thallium-201): to highlight ischaemic myocardium
- Coronary angiography: to assess coronary blood flow in diagnostically challenging cases. Occasionally gastro-oesophageal reflux disease (GORD) and chest wall disease may mimic angina.

Management

Risk factors for CAD (cigarette smoking, physical inactivity, obesity, hypertension, diabetes mellitus, hypercholesterolaemia) should be identified and corrected. Prognostic therapies for angina include:

- Aspirin: inhibits platelet aggregation by preventing the synthesis of thromboxane A_2
- Glycoprotein IIb/IIIa receptor inhibitors: prevent adherence of fibrinogen to platelets and reduce thrombus formation, and are used in 'high-risk' individuals and patients with acute coronary syndrome
- Lipid-lowering drugs (e.g. statins): have been shown to lower mortality rates in patients with CAD.

During acute episodes of angina, pain is relieved by administering oxygen, sublingual GTN and reducing anxiety. When angina occurs more frequently long-acting nitrates (isosorbide mononitrate), β-adrenergic blocking drugs (atenolol), and calcium antagonists (amlodipine) are used to reduce cardiac oxygen demands. For angina that fails to respond to medical measures, cardiac revascularisation techniques should be considered:

- Percutaneous transluminal coronary angioplasty (PTCA): stents (miniature wire coils) may be inserted into the coronary arteries to re-establish blood flow
- Coronary artery bypass grafts: to bridge severe obstructions in patients with extensive CAD.

Myocardial infarction

Myocardial infarction (MI) results from the complete occlusion (blockage) of one or more coronary arteries. It arises when atherosclerotic plaques rupture causing platelet activation, adhesion and aggregation with subsequent thrombus formation within the coronary circulation. Angina may progress to MI, but fewer than 50% of patients with MI have any preceding symptoms.

Clinical features

Myocardial infarction most commonly presents with central chest pain similar to that of angina. Unlike angina it is not relieved by rest or with sublingual nitrates. Vomiting, nausea, restlessness, sweating, shortness of breath, and a feeling of 'impending doom' are common. Approximately 10–20% of individuals have silent (painless) infarctions and the first sign may be the catastrophic onset of left ventricular failure, shock, loss of consciousness and death. Up to 50% of patients die within the first hour of MI and a further 10–20% within the next few days. Fatal cardiac arrhythmias (ventricular fibrillation), valvular dysfunction, cardiac failure and myocardial rupture may complicate an MI.

Clinical signs

- An ECG shows typical changes of an anterior inferior infarct (Figures 1.6 and 1.7).

Diagnosis

The diagnosis of an MI is based mainly on clinical features supported by characteristic ECG changes (ST segment elevation, T-wave inversion, pathological

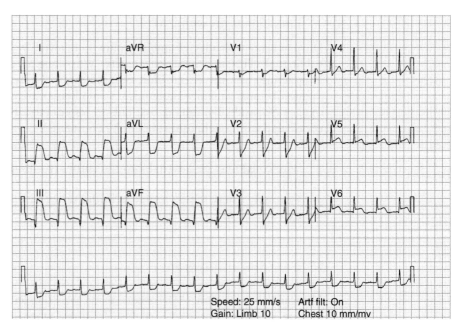

Figure 1.6 This ECG shows massive ST segment elevation in the inferior leads (II, III and aVF) with lesser elevation in the lateral chest leads (V5 and V6). There is so-called reciprocal ST depression in leads I, aVL, V2 and V3. These changes are consistent with an acute apical myocardial infarction

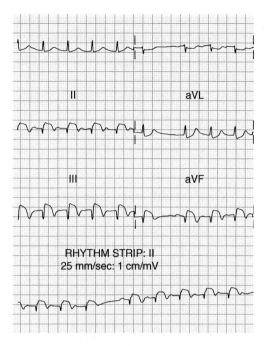

Figure 1.7 There is elevation of the ST segments in the inferior leads (II, III and aVF) along with T-wave inversion and Q wave formation. There is also prolongation of the PR interval eventually leading to a dropped beat, typical of Wenckebach phenomenon (second degree heart block). These changes indicate an acute inferior myocardial infarction

Q waves). Damaged (infarcted) cardiac muscle releases several enzymes and proteins into the circulation – troponin (an early marker of heart damage), cardiac specific creatine kinase (CK-MB), aspartate transaminase (AST) and lactate dehydrogenase (LDH). Serial blood measurements of these enzymes allows the time course of the MI to be followed.

Management

Myocardial infarction requires immediate hospital admission. Early treatment halves the mortality rate. Management aims include adequate pain relief, limitation of the extent of damage to the myocardium (infarct size) and prevention/early treatment of complications. Immediate treatment of an MI includes:

- Alert emergency services (if in community) or cardiac arrest team (if in hospital)
- Aspirin (300 mg): to be chewed
- Pain relief: opioid analgesia (diamorphine) is usually necessary
- Oxygen or nitrous oxide with at least 28% oxygen
- Thrombolytic agent (streptokinase/tissue plasminogen activator [t-PA]) to dissolve the coronary thrombus provided the patient is not at risk of a life-threatening haemorrhage
- Glyceryl trinitrate infusion to relieve pain and prevent pulmonary oedema (fluid accumulation within the lungs)

- Prompt treatment of complications, particularly cardiac arrhythmias, including the initiation of cardiopulmonary resuscitation.

Subsequent management of an MI includes initiation of secondary prevention therapy including:

- An ACE inhibitor: cardioprotective against subsequent events
- Early mobilisation
- Cardiac rehabilitation programme
- Correction of risk factors for CAD (as in the management of angina).

Oral health care relevance

- Angina can be precipitated by the stress and anxiety associated with dental treatment. Appointment times should therefore be kept as short as possible and the dental team should be empathetic and reassuring at all times.
- Preoperative oral temazepam (e.g. 10 mg at night prior to the day of the appointment and a further 10 mg on the morning of the appointment) may be helpful in reducing anxiety.
- Appointments should be scheduled to avoid early mornings as endogenous adrenaline [epinephrine] levels are higher at this time, potentially increasing the risk of adverse cardiac events.
- The use of adrenaline-containing local anaesthetics is not contraindicated. Profound anaesthesia is most important and an effective aspirating technique is necessary to avoid intravascular injections.
- Conscious sedation in the primary care setting is best avoided in patients with a recent history (6–12 months) of myocardial infarction or angina, and also in patients with unstable angina. The reader is reminded of The Department of Health's Standing Dental Advisory Committee document 'Conscious Sedation in the Provision of Dental Care, 2003'. This states that conscious sedation in the primary care setting should only be administered to patients in ASA (American Society of Anaesthesiologists) groups I and II (i.e. normal healthy individuals or a patient with systemic disease but no functional impairment).
- The patient's GTN medication should be readily available in case of an angina attack. Continuous chest pain for more than 3 minutes following its administration and giving oxygen is suggestive of a myocardial infarction. Oxygen (100%) should be continued, the patient given chewable aspirin and help summoned. 'Entonox' (1:1 nitrous oxide:oxygen) may be given to allay anxiety and provide analgesia.
- Patients with a history of myocardial infarction within the previous 6 months are regarded as being at greater risk of developing a further infarct during this time. Therefore, more complex procedures are best deferred.
- Angina can mimic dental pain spreading along the lower teeth and jaw.
- The medication of patients with ischaemic heart disease must be considered as they can cause oral manifestations (e.g. nicorandil used in the management of angina can produce severe oral ulceration). Potential drug

interactions must also be taken into account (e.g. concurrent use of triazole and imidazole anti-fungal agents should be avoided with the statins as this increases the risk of myopathy).

A stable cardiac patient receiving atraumatic treatment under local anaesthesia should be manageable in dental practice. A patient requiring complex surgery, a general anaesthetic or who is unstable with dyspnoea on minimal exertion, cyanosis, frequent angina or a recent MI, requires treatment in hospital.

Hypertension

Hypertension is a persistently raised blood pressure (BP). The BP is measured with a sphygmomanometer, in units of millimetres of mercury (mmHg). Hypertension may be defined as an elevated blood pressure of at least 140/90 mmHg, based on at least two readings on separate occasions. The BP will vary depending on age, gender, ethnicity, environment, emotional state and activity. The BP tends to increase with age but in more than 90% of people with hypertension the cause is unknown. This is termed 'primary' or 'essential' hypertension. Aetiological factors include:

- Genetic predisposition
- High alcohol intake
- High salt intake
- Smoking
- High body mass index (BMI)
- Impaired tissue response to insulin (insulin resistance)
- Sympathetic overactivity: approximately 40% of hypertensive patients have raised levels of circulating catecholamines (epinephrine [adrenaline] and norepinephrine [noradrenaline]).

In 1–2% of hypertensive patients an underlying cause is present and this is termed 'secondary' hypertension. Causes include:

- Renal disease: responsible for over 80% of cases
- Endocrine disorders
- Pregnancy
- Drugs (oral contraceptive pill)
- Narrowing of the aorta (coarctation).

Accelerated (malignant) hypertension is uncommon and seen mainly in people of African descent. It can have an acute onset or may develop in individuals with pre-existing essential hypertension. It is potentially life threatening and should be regarded as a medical emergency.

Clinical features

About 20% of the population are hypertensive with the majority being asymptomatic, and about one third of individuals being unaware that they have the condition. Longstanding hypertension accelerates atheroma (atherosclerosis) and predisposes to damage to the:

- Heart (coronary artery disease)
- Brain (cerebrovascular disease), particularly stroke
- Kidneys (chronic renal failure)
- Hands and feet, rarely (peripheral vascular disease)
- Eyes (hypertensive retinopathy), leading to blindness.

Accelerated hypertension may present with headaches, visual impairment, nausea, vomiting, fits (seizures) or acute cardiac failure.

Clinical signs

Anti-hypertensive medication can produce a variety of orofacial side effects such as gingival overgrowth from calcium channel blockers e.g. nifedipine, amlodipine (Figure 1.8).

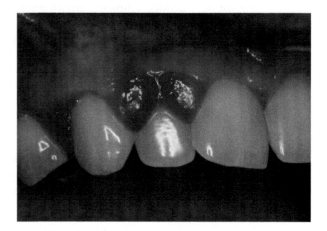

Figure 1.8   Gingival overgrowth caused by calcium channel blockers

Diagnosis

Hypertension is diagnosed by standardised serial BP measurements. Investigations to identify a 'secondary' cause and assess end-organ damage include:

- Chest radiograph: increased cardiac size (cardiomegaly) is suggestive of hypertensive heart disease
- Electrocardiogram (ECG): may indicate ischaemic heart disease and show changes of left ventricular hypertrophy
- Serum urea and electrolytes: deranged in hypertensive renal disease and endocrine causes of secondary hypertension
- Urine dipstick testing: blood and protein in the urine suggests renal disease.

Management

Treatment of hypertension reduces the risk of stroke, heart failure and renal failure. It has less of an effect on ischaemic cardiac events. General measures that lower BP include:

- Relaxation
- Smoking cessation
- Restricting alcohol intake
- Low salt diet
- High fibre diet
- Weight reduction
- Regular exercise.

A large number of drugs are currently available for the treatment of hypertension (Table 1.2).

Table 1.2 Anti-hypertensive drugs

Anti-hypertensive agents	Examples
Diuretics	Bendroflumethiazide, furosemide
Angiotensin converting enzyme (ACE) inhibitors	Enalapril, ramipril, perindopril
Angiotensinogen II receptor blockers (ARB)	Candesartan, losartan, telmisartan
β-adrenergic blockers	Atenolol, propanolol
Calcium channel blockers	Amlodipine, nifedipine
α-adrenergic blockers	Doxazosin
	Moxonidine

A single agent (monotherapy) is used initially, but combination therapy may be needed in more resistant cases for adequate control of the BP. The most effective drug combinations include:

- An ACE inhibitor with a diuretic
- An ARB with a calcium antagonist.

Life-threatening accelerated hypertension requires urgent hospital admission with the aim to reduce the BP slowly with oral anti-hypertensives. Rarely, intravenous anti-hypertensives (e.g. sodium nitroprusside) are used, but a sudden drop in BP may result in a stroke (cerebral infarction).

Oral health care relevance

- Essential hypertension is not in itself associated with orofacial manifestations. There may, however, be a plethoric facial complexion in patients with very elevated blood pressure.
- Anti-hypertensive medication can produce a variety of orofacial side effects
  - beta blockers: xerostomia and lichenoid reactions
  - calcium channel blockers: gingival overgrowth (Figure 1.8)
  - angiotensin converting inhibitors: lichenoid reactions, burning sensations of the oral mucosa
  - angiotensin II receptor blockers: lichenoid reactions, burning sensations of the oral mucosa.

- The provision of dental care should be as stress free as possible. It may be advantageous to avoid early morning appointments as this is when blood pressure is highest and adverse cardiac events more likely to occur.
- Local anaesthetics containing adrenaline (epinephrine) are not contraindicated in patients with hypertension, although it is prudent to use the minimal amount consistent with obtaining satisfactory anaesthesia. An exception is in those patients with severe (diastolic pressure greater than 140 mm/Hg) or malignant hypertension. Both of these conditions require urgent hospital referral.
- Following lengthy dental treatment in the supine position, the patient should be returned to the upright position slowly to minimise the risk of postural hypotension.
- Long term, inadequately managed hypertension may lead to cardiac, cerebrovascular and renal complications, which may in turn impact on the provision of dental treatment (see appropriate sections).

Congenital heart disease

Congenital lesions may involve the heart or adjacent great vessels either in isolation or in a variety of combinations. They are the most common type of heart disease in children and in developed countries, affecting about 1 in 1000 live births. A variety of factors may give rise to congenital heart disease (CHD). These include:

- Congenital rubella and cytomegalovirus infection
- Maternal drug and alcohol abuse
- Single gene mutations
- As a feature of hereditary syndromes (Down syndrome).

Congenital heart disease may be cyanotic – 'blue babies' (Table 1.3), where there is right-to-left shunting and in general more severe defects, or acyanotic (Table 1.4).

Clinical features

In cyanotic CHD reduced oxygen carriage (chronic hypoxaemia) leads to impaired development; polycythaemia and gross clubbing of fingers and toes may result. Patients may crouch in an attempt to improve venous return of the

Table 1.3 Cyanotic congenital heart disease (CHD)

Congenital heart lesion	Nature of defect
Transposition of the great vessels	Reversal of the origins of the pulmonary artery and aorta
Tetralogy of Fallot	Ventricular septal defect, pulmonary stenosis, right ventricular hypertrophy and an aorta that overrides both ventricles
Eisenmenger syndrome	Right to left shunting of blood flow through the heart

Table 1.4   Acyanotic congenital heart disease (CHD)

Congenital heart lesion	Nature of defect
Mitral valve prolapse (floppy mitral valve)	The most common cardiac defect, 20% of the population
Ventricular septal defect (VSD)	Common. Usually a single opening in the interventricular septum
Patent ductus arteriosus (PDA)	A persistent opening between the aorta and pulmonary artery
Pulmonary valve stenosis	Narrowing of the pulmonary valve
Atrial septal defect (ASD)	An opening in the atrial septum. Many different forms ranging from a simple primum defect to a complex atrioventricular septal defect
Coarctation of the aorta	Narrowing of the aorta usually sited beyond the origin of the subclavian arteries. The blood supply to the head, neck and upper body are normal but the circulation to the lower part of the body is restricted
Aortic valve stenosis	Narrowing of the aortic valve, most commonly secondary to a congenital bicuspid valve

blood to the heart. Both haemorrhagic and thrombotic tendencies may arise. Cyanotic congenital heart defects invariably result in heart failure, and in the absence of treatment 40% of individuals die within the first 5 years. Approximately 20% of patients with CHD have other congenital anomalies.

Clinical signs

Central cyanosis and a malar flush (Figure 1.9) can be congenital or acquired. Atrial fibrillation (AF) occurs in 40% and reactive pulmonary hypertension in 25% of patients with severe stenosis, acute pulmonary oedema, infective endocarditis, bronchitis and recurrent pulmonary embolism; the lady shown in Figure 1.9 suffers from orthopnoea and paroxysmal nocturnal dyspnoea.

Congenital mitral stenosis is usually associated with other lesions causing left ventricular outflow obstruction including atrial stenosis, subaortic stenosis, coarctation and atrial myxoma. In 99% of patients, this is acquired and due to rheumatic heart disease. Other rare causes include infective endocarditis,

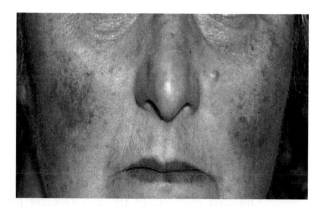

Figure 1.9   Patient with central cyanosis and a malar flush

granulomatous infiltration in association with eosinophilia, calcified mitral valve ring and systemic lupus erythematosus.

Diagnosis

- Antenatal ultrasound: allows early diagnosis
- Chest radiograph: may show cardiomegaly
- Electrocardiogram: may demonstrate an abnormal cardiac axis, ventricular hypertrophy and strain depending on the lesion present
- Echocardiography: allows the majority of defects to be diagnosed non-invasively and has now superseded intracardiac catheter studies.

Management

Early correction of the congenital defect is the treatment of choice and an increasing number of lesions are now treated by transvenous catheter techniques thereby avoiding the need for invasive surgery. More complex defects may require an operation. Although surgery has enormously improved the prognosis for patients with CHD, residual defects can predispose to infective endocarditis. Medical treatment may also be needed for the management of:

- Pulmonary oedema
- Heart failure
- Polycythaemia
- Infection
- Emotional disturbances.

Children with CHD receiving modern surgical and medical care now often survive into adult life, so-called 'grown-up' congenital heart disease.

Oral health care relevance

The National Institute for Health and Clinical Excellence (NICE) clinical guideline 64, 'Prophylaxis Against Infective Endocarditis', was published in March 2008. This stated that antibiotic prophylaxis against infective endocarditis for invasive dental procedures in patients previously considered as being 'at risk' is no longer recommended. Additionally NICE stated that chlorhexidine gluconate mouth rinses should not be offered to such patients. The recommendations of NICE are based on the lack of supporting evidence that dental treatment predisposes patients to infective endocarditis. There is also evidence that the risk of serious adverse events to antibiotics is substantially greater than the risk of causing infective endocarditis from dental procedures in 'susceptible' patients.

Infective endocarditis

Infective endocarditis (IE) is a rare but potentially life-threatening infection, predominantly affecting damaged heart valves. Platelet–fibrin deposits may form along the free margins of damaged valves, where there is turbulent blood flow. These sterile vegetations (aseptic thrombotic endocarditis) may become infected with organisms resulting in large friable vegetations. Cardiac lesions that predispose to infective endocarditis include:

- Congenital or acquired valvular defects
- Prosthetic heart valves
- Atrial and ventricular septal defects
- Patent ductus arteriosus
- Complex congenital heart disease (e.g. tetralogy of Fallot)
- Surgically constructed systemic–pulmonary shunts.

Individuals who have had uncomplicated myocardial infarcts, coronary angioplasty, coronary artery bypass grafts and cardiac pacemakers inserted do not have an increased risk of developing IE.

Oral viridans streptococci (*Streptococcus mutans* and *S. sanguis*) have complex attachment mechanisms that enable them to adhere to damaged endocardium, and they are responsible for approximately 50% of cases of IE. Viridans streptococci enter the bloodstream (bacteraemia) during tooth extractions and other oral procedures, including toothbrushing and scaling. The majority of bacteraemias are transient, self-limiting and not associated with any systemic complications. The factors that determine the development of IE are complex, but a susceptible cardiac surface (damaged endocardium) and high bacterial loads within the circulation appear to be important.

Clinical features

The clinical features of IE are highly variable, often with an insidious onset, but should be considered in any individual presenting with fever and a new or changing heart murmur. Symptoms and signs reflect:

- Progressive heart damage (valve destruction and heart failure)
- Infection (fever, malaise, night sweats and weight loss)
- Embolic damage of organs (brain, lungs, spleen and kidneys)
- Immune complex formation (leading to vasculitis, arthritis and renal and retinal damage).

Clinical signs

Splinter haemorrhages (Figure 1.10) are seen in approximately 10% of patients with infective endocarditis. Other signs may include:

- Petechial spots (small and red with a pale centre, often seen in the pharynx and conjunctivae; when present on the retina they are known as Roth spots)
- Osler nodes (hard, tender subcutaneous swellings in the hands and feet)
- Janeway lesions (small, flat, red, non-tender macules on the thenar eminences)
- Pallor (due to anaemia)
- Finger clubbing may be a late feature.

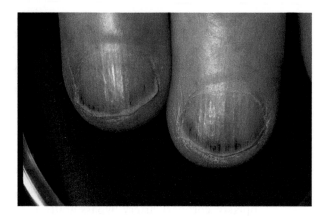

Figure 1.10   Splinter haemorrhages

Diagnosis

- Clinical history and presentation
- At least three sets of blood cultures over 24 hours before starting antibiotics
- Electrocardiogram (ECG): may show conduction abnormalities
- Echocardiography (ECHO): may identify vegetations and enables assessment of valvular and cardiac function
- Urine dipstick testing to detect microscopic haematuria
- Serological testing to identify atypical organisms (e.g. Legionella).

Management

Without treatment, IE is fatal in approximately 30% of patients, so the patient should be admitted to hospital for intravenous antibiotic therapy, usually benzylpenicillin and gentamicin. If staphylococcal endocarditis is suspected vancomycin should be substituted in place of penicillin. In severe cases, such as prosthetic valve endocarditis, early removal of the infected valve and insertion of a sterile replacement may be needed.

Patients at risk of endocarditis should receive intensive preventive dental care to minimise the need for dental intervention. In many countries there are national guidelines on the use of antimicrobial prophylaxis against IE if dental interventions are needed. Although the efficacy of such antimicrobial prophylaxis may be questionable, individuals with susceptible cardiac lesions (as outlined above) were typically given antibiotic therapy prior to undergoing procedures likely to result in bacteraemia.

- NICE no longer recommends antibiotic prophylaxis for patients with a previous history of infective endocarditis who are to receive invasive dental treatment (see also *Congenital heart disease* section).

2 Respiratory conditions

Lung cancer

- Lung cancer is the most common cancer in developed countries in males, and most frequently affects urban, adult cigarette smokers.
- Bronchogenic carcinoma accounts for most primary lung tumours.
- Metastases from cancers elsewhere are also frequent in the lungs.

Clinical features

- Main features are recurrent cough, haemoptysis, dyspnoea, chest pain and chest infections.
- Local infiltration can cause any of the following:
  - pleural effusion
  - cervical sympathetic chain lesions (Horner syndrome)
  - brachial neuritis
  - recurrent laryngeal nerve palsy
  - superior vena cava obstruction with facial cyanosis and oedema (superior vena cava syndrome).
- Metastases are common, typically to the
  - brain: headache, epilepsy, hemiplegia or visual disturbances
  - liver: hepatomegaly, jaundice or ascites
  - bone: pain, swelling or pathological fracture.
- Loss of weight, finger clubbing and anorexia are common.

Clinical signs

Finger clubbing (Figure 2.1) is diagnosed when there is loss of the angle between the nail and the nail-bed (best to examine the fingers from the side). Other features are:

- Redness and a boggy texture to the nail-bed
- Increased curvature of the nail
- Increase in the soft tissue volume of the finger ends
- Eventually the fingers can take on a drumstick-like appearance as shown.

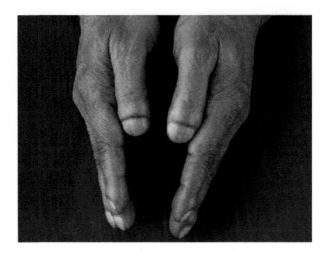

Figure 2.1   Finger clubbing

Finger clubbing has a range of causes:

- Respiratory: bronchial carcinoma, cystic fibrosis
- Gastrointestinal tract: inflammatory bowel disease (Crohn disease in particular)
- Cardiac: endocarditis, congenital cyanotic heart disease
- Others: idiopathic, familial.

Diagnosis

- Radiography, CT (spiral CT can detect early tumours) and MRI
- Sputum cytology, bronchoscopy and biopsy.

Management

- Radiotherapy is commonly used.
- The overall 5-year survival rate is only 8%.

Oral health care relevance

- Oral cancer may be associated with lung cancer, and vice versa. Tumours at these sites may either develop at similar times (synchronous) or else may develop at a later stage (metachronous).
- Metastases can occasionally affect the orofacial region, typically involving the supraclavicular lymph nodes in the later stages of the disease.
- Pigmentation of the soft palate is a rare manifestation of lung cancer, and it may occur early in the course of the disease.

The use of sedation techniques (intravenous and inhalational) should only be considered after consultation with the patient's respiratory physician who can advise on the level of residual respiratory function. Because lung cancer nearly always occurs on a background of smoking-related chronic obstructive pulmonary disease, the same considerations apply as in the section on *Chronic obstructive pulmonary disease* (p. 24).

Asthma

Asthma is a common condition and is caused by bronchial hyper-reactivity. It results in reversible airway obstruction secondary to excessive bronchial smooth muscle tone (bronchospasm), mucosal oedema and hypersecretion of mucus.

The prevalence of asthma is increasing. It is more common in males and usually begins in childhood or early adult life. Asthma has traditionally been classified into extrinsic (atopic) and intrinsic (non-atopic) disease (Table 2.1). However, it is now recognised that almost all asthmatic patients have an allergic component to their disease.

Table 2.1   Traditional classification of asthma

	Extrinsic asthma	Intrinsic asthma
Frequency	Common	Less common
Associations	Atopic disease (eczema, allergic rhinitis)	
Pathogenesis	IgE mediated mast cell degranulation	Intrinsic mast cell instability
Age of onset	Early onset Child- or early adulthood	Late onset
Precipitating factors	Allergens identified by positive skin-prick test Animal hairs House-dust mite Pollen and moulds	Air pollutants Cold air Drugs (e.g. NSAIDs) Emotional stress Exercise

NSAIDs, non-steroidal anti-inflammatory drugs.

Clinical features

In well-controlled patients clinical features may be absent. During an asthmatic episode symptoms may include dyspnoea, cough and paroxysmal expiratory wheeziness with laboured expiration. On examination patients may be distressed, anxious, tachycardic, have reduced chest expansion and be using accessory respiratory muscles to increase their ventilatory effort.

A prolonged asthmatic attack that is refractory to treatment may lead to life-threatening status asthmaticus. Failure of the patient to complete a sentence, indrawing of the intercostal muscles, a silent chest and signs of exhaustion are suggestive of an impending respiratory arrest.

Clinical signs

Use of corticosteroid inhalers may predispose to oropharyngeal candidosis (Figure 2.2).

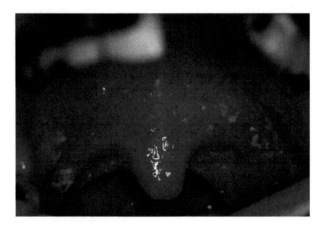

Figure 2.2   White spots indicating oropharyngeal candidosis from inhaler use

Diagnosis

Diagnosis of asthma is based on:

- Clinical history and presentation
- Serial peak expiratory flow rates (PEFRs)
- Lung function tests to assess airway reversibility
- Full blood count: may demonstrate an eosinophilia
- Serum total and specific IgE levels: raised in atopic disease
- Chest radiograph (CXR): usually normal. Important to exclude other diagnoses such as a pneumothorax, which may mimic an acute asthma attack.

Management

Management of asthma includes:

- Patient education
- PEFR diary
- Smoking cessation advice
- Avoidance of identifiable precipitants
- Pharmacotherapy (Table 2.2).

Table 2.2 Pharmacotherapy used in the management of asthma

Class of drug	Examples	Comments
Beta-2 agonists	Salbutamol, terbutaline	Safe and effective, effect lasts 3–6 hours
	Salmeterol, formoterol	Effect lasts 12 hours
Anticholinergics	Ipratropium bromide, oxitropium bromide	Effect lasts up to 8 hours
Methylxanthines	Theophylline	Prolonged duration of action
Corticosteroids	Beclometasone, fluticasone	Multiple anti-inflammatory actions
Mast cell stabilisers	Sodium cromoglicate	For prophylactic therapy
Leukotriene receptor antagonist (LTRA)	Montelukast, zafirlukast	May impair liver function

Oral health care relevance

- An acute asthmatic attack is a potential medical emergency and the clinician must be aware of its management.
- The patient's medication should be immediately available during dental treatment in case of an asthmatic attack. It is the beta-2 agonist spray (e.g. salbutamol) that should be used as an inhalation in an emergency, not the corticosteroid spray. (It is helpful to ask patients to bring all their medication with them when they attend the surgery.)
- If patients are taking oral corticosteroid therapy (e.g. prednisolone), then consideration needs to be given to steroid boosting prior to invasive dental treatment.
- The clinician should understand the precipitating factors and severity of the asthmatic attacks – anxiety is an aetiological factor in some patients and therefore a calm, reassuring approach by the dental team is most important.
- As anxiety may precipitate an asthmatic attack, a case can be made that sedation may reduce the risk of such events. However, the risk of respiratory depression from sedation techniques must be considered as this may increase the potential for respiratory failure in an acute asthmatic attack. Administration of the patient's bronchodilator prior to sedation may be a useful precaution. Most asthmatic patients are considered to fall into American Society of Anaesthesiologists group II (ASA II) and are therefore suitable for sedation within the primary care setting. However, those patients who have more than one acute asthmatic attack per week or whose attacks may respond poorly to simple therapy are classified as ASA III (a patient with systemic disease and significant functional impairment) and should be treated within a hospital setting.
- The avoidance of non-steroidal anti-inflammatory drugs including aspirin is a sensible precaution as such drugs can precipitate an asthmatic attack.
- The plasma concentration of theophylline may be increased by azithromycin.

- Oral candidosis involving the distal hard palate and soft palate is not uncommon in patients on inhaled corticosteroid medication. This can be reduced by getting the patient to rinse the mouth with water following an inhalation, or else by using spacer devices.
- There is limited evidence that patients using inhaled corticosteroids may be more prone to developing angina bullosa haemorrhagica.

Chronic obstructive pulmonary disease

Chronic obstructive pulmonary disease (COPD) is a progressive irreversible lung disease, most frequently a combination of chronic bronchitis and emphysema. Chronic bronchitis is the excessive production of mucus and persistent cough with sputum production for more than 3 months in a year for at least 2 consecutive years. It leads to excessive viscous mucus, which obstructs airways and may result in secondary chest infections commonly with *Streptococcus pneumoniae* and *Haemophilus influenzae*. Emphysema is pathological dilatation of air spaces distal to the terminal bronchioles with destruction of alveoli. The most important causes of COPD include:

- Cigarette smoking
- Environmental pollution
- Deficiency of the anti-proteolytic enzyme α-1-antitrypsin.

Clinical features

Chronic obstructive pulmonary disease is characterised by breathlessness and wheeze (airways obstruction), cough and sputum production. Progressive dyspnoea, low oxygen saturation, accumulation of carbon dioxide (hypercapnia), metabolic acidosis, respiratory failure and right sided-heart failure (cor pulmonale) may result. Patients are ultimately dyspnoeic at rest, especially when recumbent (orthopnoea). Two patterns of COPD are recognised:

- 'Pink puffers' – patients with emphysema manage to maintain normal blood gases by hyperventilation and are always breathless but not cyanosed
- 'Blue bloaters' – patients with chronic bronchitis fail to maintain adequate ventilation and become both hypercapnic and hypoxic. Chronic hypoxaemia leads to central cyanosis, cor pulmonale and oedema.

Clinical signs

Diagnosis

The diagnosis of COPD is based upon:

- Clinical history and presentation
- Chest radiography (CXR): may show hyper-inflated lung fields with loss of vascular markings (Figures 2.3 and 2.4)
- Arterial blood gases: may show evidence of either type I or type II respiratory failure

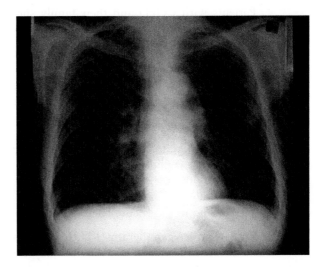

Figure 2.3 This chest x-ray shows expanded lung fields with reduced vascular lung markings and flattened diaphragms, as seen in chronic obstructive pulmonary disease

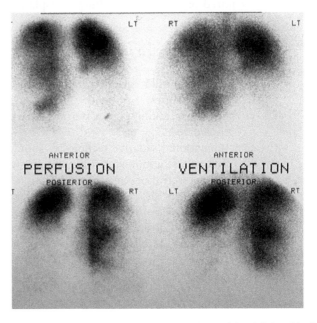

Figure 2.4 This ventilation-perfusion scan shows matching of the deficits of both lung ventilation and lung perfusion, as seen in COPD. Pulmonary embolism, in contrast, would show preserved ventilation but areas of reduced perfusion (so-called mismatched deficits)

- Spirometry and lung function tests: forced expiratory volume in 1 second (FEV1) is reduced in 80% of cases.

Management

Patients with COPD and their family should be educated about the disease, required lifestyle changes and medication. Non-drug therapy of COPD includes:

- Smoking cessation: the most important prognostic factor
- Exercise: pulmonary rehabilitation is of proven benefit
- Weight loss: improves exercise tolerance
- Vaccination: patients should receive pneumococcal and influenza vaccine.

Drug treatment of COPD includes:

- Bronchodilators: anticholinergic drugs (ipratropium bromide) and β_2-agonists (salbutamol) may be used to treat the reversible component of airway disease
- Corticosteroids (inhaled or systemic)
- Antibiotics: for acute bacterial exacerbations of COPD.

Long-term oxygen therapy (LTOT) has been shown to reduce patient mortality in COPD if given for 19 hours per day every day at a flow rate of 1–3 L/min to maintain arterial oxygen saturation above 90%. Controlled oxygen administration is needed in COPD patients to avoid causing a respiratory arrest. Advanced COPD is occasionally treated with surgery by excision of large acquired bullae or, rarely, lung transplantation.

Oral health care relevance

- Patients should not be treated fully supine as this may increase their breathing difficulties.
- For those taking corticosteroids, the need for steroid boosting should be considered.
- Inhalational sedative techniques should be avoided and intravenous sedation is best administered within a hospital setting.
- The prescription and administration of any drugs that are respiratory depressants should also be avoided where possible – this includes intravenous sedation with benzodiazepines.
- Oral candidosis may complicate the use of inhaled corticosteroids (see section on *Asthma*, p. 21).

3

Metabolic and endocrine conditions

Pregnancy

- Pregnancy affects the endocrine, cardiovascular and haematological systems, and often attitude, mood or behaviour.
- Sex hormones, prolactin and thyroid hormones rise in pregnancy, but luteinising hormone (LH) and follicle stimulating hormone (FSH) levels fall. Consequences may include:
    - Deepened pigmentation, particularly of the nipples and sometimes the face (chloasma) or elsewhere (melasma)
    - Glycosuria and impaired glucose tolerance
    - Rise in both blood volume and cardiac output, associated with tachycardia.
- Medical complications can include:
    - Hypertension: may be asymptomatic but, when associated with oedema and proteinuria (pre-eclampsia), may culminate in eclampsia (hypertension, oedema, proteinuria and convulsions) which may be fatal and hazard the foetus
    - Blood hypercoagulability: can lead to venous thrombosis
    - Diabetes
    - Anaemia
    - Supine hypotension syndrome: patients become hypotensive if laid supine and the gravid uterus compresses the inferior vena cava.
- Foetal development during the first 3 months (trimester) of pregnancy is especially at risk. Most developmental defects are of unknown aetiology but, in addition to hereditary influences, infections, alcohol, smoking, drugs and irradiation can sometimes be implicated.

Clinical signs

A zone of hyperpigmentation may occur, usually on the face, involving the temple, forehead or cheeks, also known as chloasma or the 'mask of pregnancy'. Seen also in some young women taking birth control pills, melasma may rarely occur on the forearms (Figure 3.1). It is thought that oestrogen contributes to the development of melasma in predisposed persons, but it is not

27

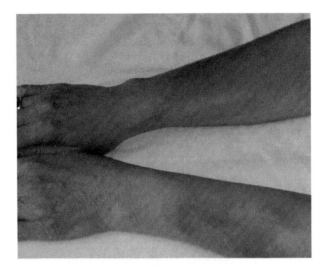

Figure 3.1   Skin hyperpigmentation on the forearms: melasma

essential to its development as men may also be affected, particularly those who use aftershave lotions or scented soaps. In pregnancy, as hormone levels return to normal after birth the hyperpigmentation often fades but will subsequently recur during the next pregnancy. Dermal melasma responds poorly to treatment although it may be of great cosmetic concern, and treatment is based on a triad of sun block, bleaching agents and patience! It can take up to 6 months to complete the process.

Pregnancy may predispose to gingivitis and associated inflammatory hyperplasias (pyogenic granulomas), often termed 'pregnancy epulides' (Figure 3.2). These may need to be removed after pregnancy.

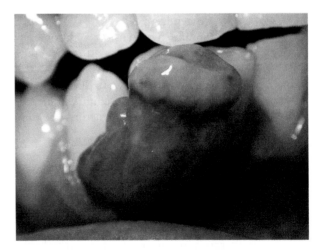

Figure 3.2   Pregnancy epulis

Oral health care relevance

- Oral manifestations of pregnancy include gingivitis and pregnancy epulis. Pregnancy may temporarily prevent recurrent aphthous stomatitis in those susceptible to this condition.
- The patient should be protected as far as possible from infections, radiography and drugs (Table 3.1).
- Inhalational and intravenous sedative techniques are best avoided during pregnancy due to possible teratogenic effects and the potential sedative effects on the foetus, general anaesthetics likewise.
- Radiography should be avoided especially in the first trimester, even though dental radiography is unlikely to be a significant risk unless the beam is directed at the foetus such as in vertex-occlusal radiography.
- As much elective dental treatment as possible should be postponed until after parturition.
- Dental treatment is best carried out during or after the second trimester.
- Elective dental care should be avoided in the last month of pregnancy, as it is uncomfortable for the patient. If treatment is necessary at this stage of pregnancy, the patient should not be treated fully supine as this may compromise venous return.
- Extensive research has failed to establish any links between amalgam usage and systemic disease in pregnancy.

Table 3.1 Drugs used in dentistry, best avoided in pregnant mothers

Drug	Potential effects on foetus
Aciclovir (systemic)	? teratogenesis
Aspirin	Bleeding tendency
	Persistent pulmonary hypertension
	Possible abortion
	Premature closure of ductus arteriosus
Carbamazepine	Neural tube defects
	Vitamin K impairment and bleeding tendency
Codeine phosphate	Respiratory depression
Corticosteroids	Adrenal suppression
	Growth retardation
Diazepam	Cleft lip/palate
Felypressin	Oxytocic
Fluconazole	Congenital anomalies
Nitrous oxide (repeated large doses)	Congenital anomalies
NSAIDs	Bleeding tendency
	Persistent pulmonary hypertension
	Premature closure of ductus arteriosus
Prilocaine	Methaemoglobinaemia
Tetracyclines	Discoloured teeth and bones
Vancomycin	Toxicity (monitor levels)

NSAIDs, non-steroidal anti-inflammatory drugs.

Breast cancer

Breast cancer is common. The causes are not clear but most cases are seen over the age of 50 years, and risk factors include:

- Genetic factors
  - Personal history of breast cancer
  - Positive family history
  - Genes (*BRCA1*, *BRCA2*, and others)
- Oestrogen exposure
  - Early menarche (onset of menstrual periods)
  - Long-term use of combined oral contraceptives or hormone replacement therapy (HRT)
  - Late childbearing
- Mutagen exposure
  - Radiation therapy
  - Alcohol
  - Smoking
- Lifestyle
  - A fatty diet
  - Obesity
  - Higher socioeconomic status.

Clinical features

Early cancer appears as a breast lump or thickening. Later, cancer may cause a change in breast size or shape, nipple discharge, tenderness or inversion, ridging or pitting (the skin looks like orange skin – 'peau d'orange') or a change in the way the skin of the breast, areola, or nipple looks or feels (e.g. warm, swollen, red or scaly).

Clinical signs

Breast cancer if advanced can fungate (Figure 3.3).

Diagnosis

Diagnosis is suggested by mammograms and often ultrasonography. Biopsy is generally needed – by needle or open biopsy.

Management

- *Lobular carcinoma in situ* (LCIS; abnormal cells in the lining of a lobule) is usually treated with tamoxifen, a hormone receptor blocker. Anastrozole is a safer alternative drug in respect of stroke risk.

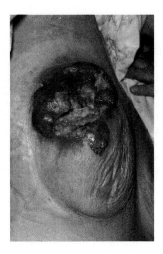

Figure 3.3 Fungation of breast cancer

- *Ductal carcinoma in situ* (DCIS or intraductal carcinoma; abnormal cells in the lining of a duct that are at risk of invasive breast cancer) is often treated with breast-sparing surgery followed by radiotherapy.
- *Breast carcinoma* is usually treated by a wide local excision with axillary node sampling or sentinel node biopsy. Histopathology results then dictate further treatment, which may be more radical surgery, or adjuvant radiotherapy sometimes plus chemotherapy. Tamoxifen is the most commonly used anti-oestrogen therapy. Treatment may include biological therapy. Trastuzumab – a monoclonal antibody that targets cells having excess human epidermal growth factor receptor-2 (HER-2) – may be given alone or along with chemotherapy.

The crude 5-year survival rate for breast cancer is now approximately 80%.

Oral health care relevance

Metastases from breast cancer occasionally affect the jaws.

Diabetes mellitus

Diabetes mellitus (DM) is a leading cause of death and disability. It affects about 4% of the general population but is recognised in only 50% of those individuals. It is more common in older persons and those of origins in the Asian subcontinent.

Diabetes mellitus is caused by a relative lack of insulin as a result of decreased production of insulin from the beta cells of the pancreatic islets of Langerhans or from increased resistance to insulin by peripheral tissues (Table 3.2). Type 2 (non-insulin dependent, maturity onset) diabetes accounts for 80–90% of patients with DM.

In DM, glucose utilisation is impaired, so it accumulates in the blood (hyperglycaemia) and the urine (glucosuria) producing an osmotic diuresis leading to

Table 3.2 Classification of diabetes mellitus

Primary	*Type 1 (insulin dependent [IDDM], juvenile onset)*
	Commonly presents before third decade. Associated with other organ-specific autoimmune diseases and characterised by antibodies against insulin and islets of Langerhans
	Type 2 (non-insulin dependent [NIDDM], maturity onset)
	Generally presents in genetically predisposed individuals over the age of 40 who are overweight. Patients develop abnormal beta cell function and resistance to insulin
Secondary	Drugs (e.g. corticosteroids, thiazide diuretics, anti-psychotics)
	Endocrine disorders (e.g. acromegaly, Cushing syndrome)
	Pancreatic disease (e.g. pancreatitis)
	Pregnancy (e.g. gestational diabetes)

the production of large volumes of urine (polyuria). As glucose is no longer a viable energy source, fat and protein stores are metabolised – with weight loss, peripheral muscle wasting and the production of ketone bodies (acetoacetate, hydroxybutyrate and acetone). These accumulate in the blood (ketonaemia) and are excreted in the urine (ketonuria). The resultant metabolic ketoacidosis leads to a compensatory increase in respiratory rate (hyperventilation) and a secondary respiratory alkalosis. In severe decompensation, ketone bodies may be detected on the breath (in particular acetone).

Clinical features

Patients with diabetes may present in a variety of ways:

- Asymptomatic: detected on routine or opportunistic screening
- Acute/chronic: presentations are related to severity and degree of onset (Table 3.3)
- Complications arise from long-term microvascular and macrovascular disease that can affect almost every part of the body (Table 3.4). Diabetes mellitus is a multisystem disorder.

Table 3.3 Acute and chronic presenting features of diabetes mellitus

Acute presenting features	Chronic presenting features
Polyuria	Polyuria
Thirst and polydipsia	Polydipsia
Dehydration	Dehydration
Ketoacidosis	Weight loss
Weight loss and weakness	Lethargy and irritability
Lethargy and irritability	Recurrent skin and genital infections
Confusion and behavioural changes	Visual deterioration
Nausea and vomiting	Paraesthesia (feet)
Abdominal pain	
Renal failure	
Coma	

Table 3.4 Micro- and macrovascular complications of diabetes mellitus

Microvascular complications	Macrovascular complications
Nephropathy	Cerebrovascular disease
Neuropathy	Coronary artery disease
Retinopathy	Hypertension
	Peripheral vascular disease

Clinical signs

Diabetic retinopathy is a serious complication (Figure 3.4).

Insulin injections may cause lipoatrophy (Figure 3.5)

Diabetes most commonly leads to peripheral vascular disease and gangrene (Figure 3.6), rarely to necrobiosis (Figure 3.7).

Less than 1% of diabetics have necrobiosis (necrobiosis lipoidica diabeticorum), but most patients with necrobiosis will have diabetes. The association is with both type 1 and type 2 diabetes and can precede the condition. It affects all races and can occur at any age, but most commonly starts between the ages of 30 and 40 years. It is three times as common in women as in men.

Necrobiosis is a disorder of collagen degeneration with a granulomatous response, thickening of blood vessel walls and fat deposition. The exact cause is unknown, but diabetic microangiopathic changes may be implicated. Other theories suggest trauma or inflammatory or metabolic alteration. It is also possible that an antibody-mediated vasculitis may cause the changes seen.

The disease is typically chronic with variable progression and scarring. Squamous cell cancers have been reported in older lesions related to previous trauma and ulceration.

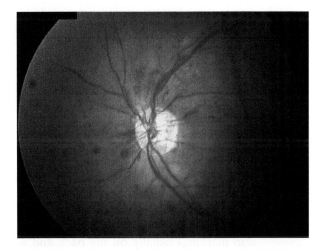

Figure 3.4 Diabetic retinopathy with leashes of new blood vessels at the optic disc

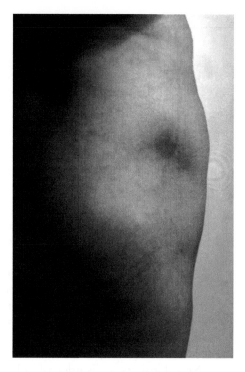

Figure 3.5   Indentation due to lipoatrophy at the site of insulin injection

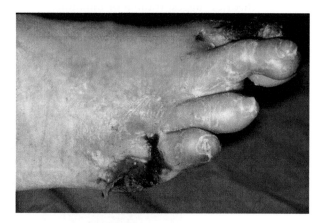

Figure 3.6   Gangrene resulting from diabetes

Trophic ulceration may also be seen in DM, because of the peripheral neuropathy (Figure 3.8).

Another skin complication is acanthosis nigricans (AN; Figure 3.9), a rare disorder that causes light-brown-to-black, velvety, rough areas or increased skin markings usually on the back and sides of the neck. The condition can also at times occur under the arms and in the groin, and in the mouth.

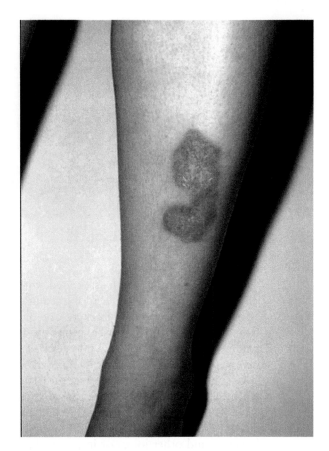

Figure 3.7   Necrobiosis lipoidica diabeticorum

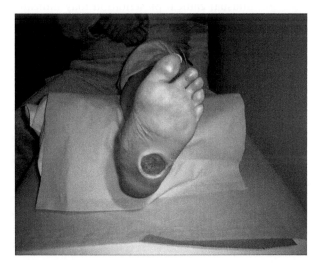

Figure 3.8   Trophic ulcer resulting from diabetes

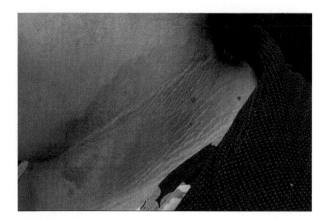

Figure 3.9   Acanthosis nigricans

Acanthosis nigricans is associated with obesity and is caused by hyper-insulinaemia, a consequence of insulin resistance. It is most common in African-Americans. The hyperkeratotic plaques of the elbows, knees and scalp may be easily confused with psoriasis, but AN can be differentiated since plaques are not inflamed, while psoriasis plaques are typically red. Classic involvement of AN in the axillae may be confirmatory.

Granuloma annulare (GA; Figure 3.10) is a common condition associated with diabetes, necrobiosis lipoidica diabeticorum, rheumatoid nodules, endocrine disorders, malignancy, HIV/AIDS and herpes zoster. It is predominantly a disease of healthy children and young adults and appears most often over knuckles and other joints or in places that are subject to frequent, mild injury such as the back of the hands or top of the feet.

Although no definite patterns relating GA and systemic disease have been thoroughly established, it has been suggested that an atypical histological or unusual clinical presentation may indicate an associated disease.

This condition is usually self-limiting and clears within 2 years.

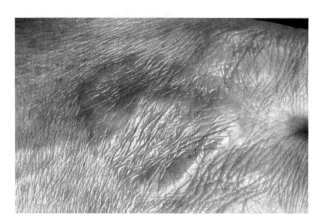

Figure 3.10   Granuloma annulare

Diabetic cheiroarthropathy is a term used to describe limited joint mobility in the hand – also termed diabetic hand syndrome, stiff hand syndrome or digital scleroderma (Figure 3.11).

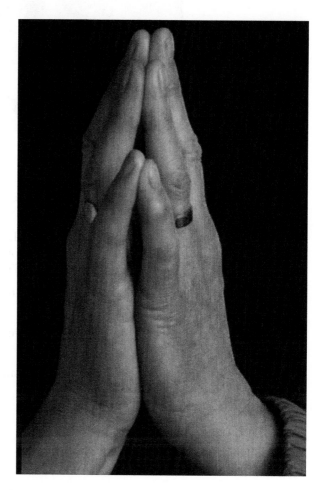

Figure 3.11   Diabetic cheiroarthropathy

Onychogryphosis describes the excessive thickening, hooking and curving of fingernails or toenails (Figure 3.12), which can be caused by several factors including diabetes, poor blood supply, infection, injuries or the inadequate intake of nutrients.

Diagnosis

Diagnosis of diabetes is from the presence of raised blood (venous plasma) glucose. The fasting plasma glucose is the preferred test.

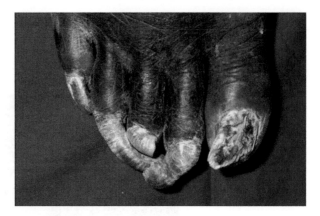

Figure 3.12   Onychogryphosis

Diabetes mellitus is confirmed when the:

- Fasting blood glucose is ≥7.0 mmol/L
- Random blood glucose is ≥11.1 mmol/L
- Blood glucose is ≥11.1 mmol/L two hours after a 75 g oral glucose challenge – oral glucose tolerance test (OGTT).

Patients are said to have impaired glucose tolerance (IGT) when:

- Fasting blood glucose is <6.1 mmol/L
- Blood glucose is 7.8–11.0 mmol/L two hours after a 75 g oral glucose challenge.

Patients with IGT may develop diabetes, and they have an increased risk of cardiovascular disease.

Management

Treatment objectives in diabetes are:

- Prevention of acute complications, especially hypoglycaemia (low blood glucose <3.0 mmol/L)
- Maintenance of near normal blood glucose levels
- Prevention of chronic complications.

Individuals should be educated with regard to the importance of good long-term diabetic control and have a thorough knowledge of the disease. The progressive nature of DM, its complications and management aims should be well understood. Patients should also be aware of the range of diabetic services available and how to make appropriate use of them. A multidisciplinary team approach is required for the effective management of diabetic individuals.

Meals should be at regular intervals, with a high fibre and relatively high carbohydrate content. Simple sugars should be avoided. An individual's calorific intake should match the person's amount of physical activity.

The efficacy of the diet is monitored by checking the weight and blood glucose levels regularly. A glucometer allows glucose readings to be taken easily by the patient at home.

The basic requirement for the treatment of type 1 diabetes is insulin administration subcutaneously, the amount being balanced against food intake and daily activities. Blood glucose levels must be monitored and used to guide the insulin dosing regimen. Insulin-treated patients are liable to hypoglycaemia due to an imbalance between food intake and insulin therapy. *Hypoglycaemic coma is a medical emergency* and may result from one or more of the following:

- Omission of a meal
- Overdosage of insulin
- Excessive exercise
- Alcohol intake.

Hypoglycaemic coma is of rapid onset and may resemble fainting. The patient may be anxious and irritable before becoming disorientated and losing consciousness. Increased sympathetic activity results in sweating, an increased heart rate (tachycardia) and pallor.

Hypoglycaemia must be quickly corrected with glucose or else brain damage can result. If the patient is conscious, a glucose solution or gel by mouth can be given. In unconscious patients 10–20 mL of 20–50% dextrose solution should be administered intravenously or, if venous access is difficult, 1 mg of glucagon intramuscularly may be given. Once conscious the patient should be given glucose orally and medical help obtained.

The basic requirement for the treatment of type 2 diabetes is controlled eating, physical activity and home blood glucose testing with a glucometer. Oral hypoglycaemic drugs may also be needed, including one or more of the following:

- Biguanides (metformin): decrease target tissue insulin resistance
- Sulphonylureas (gliclazide): increase insulin secretion
- Alpha-glucosidase inhibitors (acarbose): impair intestinal glucose absorption
- Thiazolidinediones (rosiglitazone): potentiate the action of insulin on adipose tissue
- Gliptins (sitagliptin and vildagliptin): enhance insulin secretion in response to food intake.

Long-term assessment of glucose control is made by estimation of the blood level of glycosylated haemoglobin (HbA1c), which acts as a cumulative index of control over the preceding 2–3 months.

Oral health care relevance

- The main implications of DM in dental management include:
  - Recognition and management of coma

- Glycaemic control
- Management of the sequelae (e.g. infection, cardiovascular and renal disease)
- Oral manifestations.
- The particular implications will depend upon the nature and degree of control of the diabetes.
- Dental appointments are best made in the morning, avoiding conflicts with breakfast and lunchtimes. Prior to treatment, patients should be questioned as to whether they have eaten and taken their medication as usual. If there is any uncertainty, blood glucose levels should be checked with reagent strips.
- Local anaesthesia and conscious sedation do not usually pose any risks in the diabetic patient.
- The well-controlled or moderately well-controlled diabetic patient does not pose a significant additional risk of infection following minor oral surgical procedures. It is therefore inappropriate to give such patients prophylactic antibiotic cover.
- Dental sepsis may, however, spread very rapidly. This can contribute to destabilisation of control of blood sugar leading to further worsening of the infection. Dental sepsis must be treated quickly and aggressively as it is potentially much more serious than in a non-diabetic patient. Patients should be monitored closely following surgical procedures for the possible development of infection or poor wound healing.
- Systemic corticosteroids such as prednisolone exacerbate hyperglycaemia.
- Oral manifestations of diabetes include:
  - Infections
    - Periodontal disease, including multiple lateral periodontal abscesses
    - Unusually virulent orofacial infections – should raise suspicion that the patient may have undiagnosed diabetes
    - Oral candidosis, including angular stomatitis, which may be the presenting feature
  - Xerostomia, as a result of dehydration
  - Neurological involvement
    - Burning mouth sensations, although most cases of burning mouth syndrome are unrelated to diabetes.
    - Painless, bilateral swelling of the salivary glands (sialosis) may be caused by autonomic neuropathy
  - There is debate as to whether diabetes mellitus and hypertension are related to lichen planus (Grinspan syndrome). The association may just be coincidental with commonly occurring conditions occurring together. Equally it may be related to the drugs used in these conditions, e.g. oral hypoglycaemic agents such as metformin and sulphonylureas may provoke oral lichenoid reactions in susceptible individuals.

Alcoholism

- Alcohol (ethanol) is the most common drug of abuse.

- Alcohol consumption is rising in many parts of the world.
- Alcohol effects are dose-related.
- Alcohol is a central nervous system (CNS) depressant, eventually interfering with brain higher centres, affecting judgment and concentration and cerebellar function, causing ataxia and motor in-coordination and unconsciousness.
- Alcohol use, therefore, frequently leads to trauma from accidents or assaults.
- Alcohol, after a large binge, can also suppress the cough reflex leading to vomit inhalation and death.
- Alcohol *safe maximum* daily consumption is regarded as 3–4 units for a man, 2–3 for a woman.
- Alcohol misuse (alcoholism) is consumption of alcohol to such a degree as to cause deterioration in social behaviour, or physical illness, and the development of dependence, from which withdrawal is difficult or causes adverse effects.
- Alcoholism is suggested by findings which include:
  - Social history:
    - Absenteeism
    - Assaults
    - Violence
    - Frequent job changes
    - Marital disharmony
    - Family history of alcoholism
  - Medical history:
    - Injuries (including maxillofacial) from accidents and assaults
    - Liver disease: alcoholic hepatitis and cirrhosis
    - Nutritional defects: red blood cell macrocytosis
    - Pancreatic disease: pancreatitis
    - Gastrointestinal disease: gastritis and peptic ulcer
    - Heart disease: cardiomyopathy
    - Hypertension
    - Muscle disease: myopathy
    - Brain damage and epilepsy
    - Infections, especially pneumonia and tuberculosis
    - Impaired wound healing
    - Impaired haemostasis
    - Late signs or symptoms include palpitations and tachycardia, cardiomyopathy, liver disease, malnutrition, peripheral neuropathy, amnesia and confabulation (in Wernicke and Korsakoff CNS syndromes), cerebellar degeneration with ataxia, or dementia.

Clinical signs

An enlarged purplish nose (rhinophyma) may be seen in some chronic alcoholics (Figure 3.13). This is caused by rosacea, a granulomatous condition that affects mostly caucasians of mainly north-western European descent ('curse of the Celts'); alcoholism aggravates the condition.

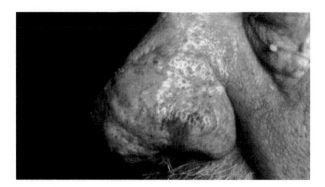

Figure 3.13 Rhinophyma due to alcoholism

Alcoholics are at risk from malnutrition, mainly because of their dietary habits. Deficiencies of B vitamins (folate, thiamine) may be seen and occasionally vitamin C deficiency (scurvy; Figure 3.14). Others at risk of chronic malnutrition include older men who live alone and the homeless, people with monotonous or odd diets, patients undergoing dialysis, people with malabsorption syndromes, inflammatory bowel disease, Whipple disease, or dyspepsia where they avoid acidic foods, or infants fed evaporated or condensed milk formulas. Scurvy produces characteristic perifollicular haemorrhages as well as corkscrew hairs, haematologic, joint, and cardiac complications. Prolonged deficiency of vitamin C intake results in defective collagen synthesis, tissue repair, and synthesis of lipids and proteins. Gingival swelling and haemorrhage commonly occur.

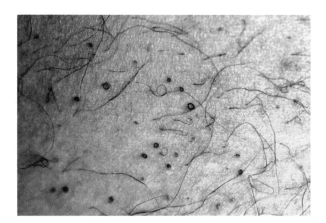

Figure 3.14 Corkscrew hairs seen in a case of scurvy

Dupuytren contractures (Figure 3.15) has long been regarded as a manifestation of alcoholism, textbooks noting associations with chronic liver disease (e.g. alcoholic cirrhosis), diabetes, epilepsy, HIV and occupations that involve repetitive trauma to the palms (e.g. lorry drivers). However, probably the

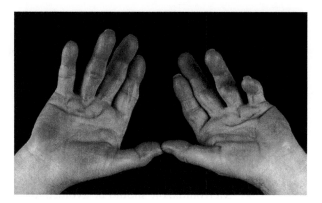

Figure 3.15 Dupuytren contractures

strongest aetiological factor is genetic: a family history of the condition is common and this is often blamed on the Viking race, as patients tend to be blue-eyed Northern Europeans.

Initially there is usually a palmar nodule in the line of the ring or small finger. This is painless but progresses to a flexion contracture affecting the fingers. Limitation of mobility is the major issue; this can lead to patients poking themselves in the eye whilst washing their face. If the contracture is severe then the finger nail will impinge on the palm and may cause ulceration.

Diagnosis

- A positive response to any of the questions in the CAGE questionnaire suggests a diagnosis of alcoholism:
  - Have you ever felt the need to Cut down on drink?
  - Have you ever felt Annoyed by criticism of your drinking?
  - Have you ever felt Guilty about drinking?
  - Do you drink a morning Eye opener?
- Helpful investigations may include red cell macrocytosis, folate and thiamine deficiency of no obvious cause and raised blood levels of:
  - alcohol
  - carbohydrate deficient transferrin
  - gamma-glutamyl transpeptidase (GGT or gamma GT) and other liver enzymes.

Management

- Admission for rehabilitation and to ensure abstinence.
- Nutritional replacement for missing folate and thiamine etc.
- Medication to reduce dependence (naltrexone, acamprosate or chlormethiazole).

Oral health care relevance

- There is a relationship between alcohol consumption and oral cancer and potentially malignant disorders.
- Treatment challenges may include:
  - Erratic attendance
  - Aggressive behaviour
  - Poly-substance misuse
  - Smoking
  - Bleeding tendency.
- Aspirin should be avoided as it may cause gastric erosions and bleeding.
- Metronidazole should be avoided due to its interaction with alcohol, which can cause widespread vasodilatation, nausea, vomiting, sweating and headache.
- Careful titration of intravenous sedatives is required as the effects are unpredictable, being dependent on the degree of liver damage and function (see section on *Chronic liver disease*, below).
- Painless swelling of the salivary glands, usually parotids, may occur in some patients with chronic alcoholism (sialosis).
- Dental erosion may be caused directly by alcohol, or from gastric regurgitation.

Chronic liver disease

Chronic liver disease or cirrhosis is characterised by the replacement of normal functioning liver with dysfunctional fibrotic tissue and regenerating nodules of hepatocytes. Approximately 30% of cases are idiopathic whilst excessive alcohol intake, viral hepatitis and drug-induced liver damage account for most of the remaining cases. Rare causes include: haemochromatosis, Wilson disease (copper deposition) and autoimmune primary biliary cirrhosis.

Clinical features

The clinical features of liver disease depend upon the nature, extent and chronicity of the underlying pathology. The liver has a central role in many important metabolic pathways, especially metabolism (e.g. bilirubin, hormones, glucose and drugs) and blood clotting factor production. The clinical manifestations therefore reflect disturbed function of these processes and include:

- Jaundice (caused by raised serum bilirubin)
- Impaired drug handling
- Hypoglycaemia
- Hepatic encephalopathy
- Gynaecomastia
- Testicular atrophy
- Bruising and haemorrhage.

Other features may include palmar erythema, pruritus, spider naevi, leuconychia, finger clubbing, recurrent infection, ascites, distended abdominal veins, hepatomegaly and a tremor (liver flap).

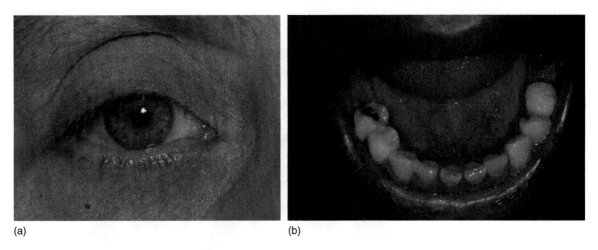

(a)   (b)

Figure 3.16   Jaundice showing in (a) the sclera and (b) the mouth

Clinical signs

Jaundice may be seen in the sclerae or occasionally the mouth (Figure 3.16a and b).

Spider naevi (Figure 3.17). – so called because they look like spiders – are telangiectasia having a central arteriole with small vessels radiating outwards. Compression of the central vessel causes the spider to disappear, only to return (via central filling) when the pressure is released. Spider naevi are only found in the distribution of the superior vena cava (i.e. above the nipple line) but the reason for this is unknown. They are a sign of chronic liver disease, more than five being regarded as pathological. These signs may be seen in patients with primary biliary cirrhosis. Such patients frequently have dry mouth as a consequence of concomitant Sjögren syndrome. Oral lichen planus may be associated with liver disease such as primary biliary cirrhosis and chronic active hepatitis.

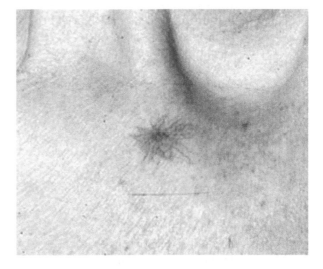

Figure 3.17   Spider naevi

Parotid gland swelling may occur as a result of alcoholic sialosis (see Figure 6.3).

Palmar erythema (Figure 3.18) describes the redness of the skin of the palms (and, in this case, the fingers) seen in chronic liver disease ('liver palms'), rheumatoid arthritis, systemic lupus erythematosus (SLE), bronchial carcinoma and in states of high cardiac output (e.g. pregnancy or thyrotoxicosis).

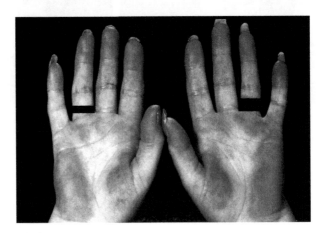

Figure 3.18   Palmar erythema

Diagnosis

The diagnosis of liver disease depends upon the history, clinical findings and targeted investigations to ascertain the nature of the underlying pathological process. Referral to a hepatologist or gastroenterologist is generally appropriate. Investigations include:

- Full blood count
- Liver function tests including coagulation studies
- Serum biochemistry (bilirubin; liver enzymes such as aspartate transaminase)
- Hepatitis viral serology
- Liver ultrasound
- Abdominal computed tomography (CT) or magnetic resonance imaging (MRI)
- Liver biopsy.

Management

The management of patients with chronic liver disease is complicated but the main points are:

- Patient education
- Alcohol reduction or cessation
- Dietary modification

- Fluid and electrolyte balance
- Awareness and correction of coagulation abnormalities
- Banding of oesophageal varices and management of portal hypertension to reduce the risk of catastrophic gastrointestinal haemorrhage
- Careful drug prescribing in view of impaired drug handling and an increased risk of drug toxicity
- Treatment of underlying viral disease (hepatitis B)
- Prevention and aggressive treatment of infection to reduce the risk of developing overwhelming sepsis.

Oral health care relevance

The major implications of chronic liver disease in dentistry relate to:

- Abnormal drug metabolism: caution must be exercised when prescribing drugs.
  - Some drugs should be avoided (Table 3.5).
  - Lower doses than usual may be required, dependent on the nature and severity of the liver disease and the drug to be prescribed.
  - Intravenous sedation must be administered cautiously as its pharmacological effects may be unpredictable. Either over- or under-sedation may result dependent on the level of functional impairment of the liver.

Table 3.5 Drug use in liver disease

Drugs to be avoided or used with caution in patients with liver disease	Alternative drugs
Analgesics	
Aspirin	Codeine
NSAIDS	COX-2 inhibitors
Opioids	
Paracetamol	
Antimicrobials	
Aminoglycosides	Penicillins
Metronidazole	Cephalosporins
Clindamycin	Tetracyclines
Co-amoxiclav	Minocycline
Doxycycline	
Imidazole and triazole anti-fungals	Polyene anti-fungals [nystatin or amphotericin]
Sedatives	
Diazepam	Lorazepam/oxazepam.
Midazolam	

NSAIDs, non-steroidal anti-inflammatory drugs.

- An additional complication of chronic liver disease may be that of hypoalbuminaemia, leading to less protein-bound drug, and therefore increased free drug in the circulation, resulting in an enhanced pharmacological effect.
- It is important to seek guidance from the British National Formulary prior to prescribing to patients with chronic liver disease.
- It is also sensible to avoid non-steroidal anti-inflammatory drugs including aspirin because of their tendency to promote gastric bleeding.
- Potential haemorrhage as a consequence of deranged synthesis of the Vitamin K-dependent clotting factors and, in some cases, an associated thrombocytopaenia. It is prudent to undertake a preoperative coagulation screen and platelet count. If the results indicate a potential haemorrhagic risk, referral for appropriate management is required.
- Cross-infection implications (mainly hepatitis B or C).
- Orofacial manifestations of chronic liver disease include:
  - Sjögren syndrome secondary to primary biliary cirrhosis. There is limited evidence that hepatitis C may also be associated with Sjögren syndrome.
  - Lichen planus secondary to chronic active hepatitis or primary biliary cirrhosis and hepatitis C in certain populations (notably Japanese and Mediterranean peoples).

Chronic kidney disease

Diabetes mellitus is the single most common cause of chronic kidney disease (CKD) in westernised countries. Other causes include:

- Hypertension: hypertensive nephropathy
- Renal artery stenosis
- Chronic glomerulonephritis (amyloidosis, lupus erythematosus)
- Drugs that are nephrotoxic (e.g. non-steroidal anti-inflammatory drugs)
- Urinary tract obstruction causing reflux nephropathy
- Nephrocalcinosis secondary to tuberculosis
- Hereditary polycystic kidney disease
- Malignancy (myeloma).

An international classification of CKD has identified five stages (stages 1–3 are early CKD; Table 3.6). Stages 1 and 2 are characterised by structural abnormalities, with persistent proteinuria or albuminuria or haematuria. Stage 3 is characterised by impaired function as defined by estimated glomerular filtration rate (eGFR) of 30–59 mL/min/1.73 m^2 on at least two occasions at a minimal interval of 3 months. When greater than 90% of renal function has been lost the term end-stage renal failure (ESRF) is used.

Chronic kidney disease causes significant impairment of renal function, which eventually affects virtually all body systems, resulting in

- Hypertension
- Deranged serum biochemistry as potassium and hydrogen ions accumulate

Table 3.6 Stages of chronic kidney disease

Stage	eGFR (mL/min/1.73m^2)	Description
1	>90	Normal or increased GFR, with other evidence of kidney damage
2	60–89	Slight decrease in GFR, with other evidence of kidney damage
3	30–59	Moderate decrease in GFR, with or without other evidence of kidney damage
4	15–29	Severe decrease in GFR, with or without other evidence of kidney damage
5	<15	Established renal failure

eGFR, estimated glomerular filtration rate

- Renal osteodystrophy: phosphate retention depresses plasma calcium levels resulting in secondary hyperparathyroidism. Deficient renal production of 1,25-dihydroxycholecalciferol (vitamin D3) leads to reduced calcium absorption
- Anaemia: renal production of erythropoietin is impaired
- Haemorrhagic tendency: platelet function is impaired giving rise to purpura and widespread bruising
- Increased risk of infection: due to defective phagocyte function and altered immune function.

Clinical features

The clinical features of CKD are diverse and are shown in Table 3.7.

Clinical signs

Haemodialysis access is facilitated by an arteriovenous fistula created surgically by connecting an artery to a vein, usually below the elbow. The increased pressure on the venous wall causes the vein to enlarge, although the degree of dilatation shown in Figure 3.19 is unusual.

Table 3.7 The clinical features of chronic kidney disease (CKD)

System	Manifestation
Cardiovascular	Hypertension, congestive cardiac failure, cardiomyopathy, pericarditis, peripheral vascular disease
Endocrine	Impotence, amenorrhoea, infertility
Gastrointestinal	Anorexia, nausea, vomiting, peptic ulcer disease, haemorrhage, diarrhoea
Haematological	Anaemia, lymphopaenia, haemorrhage, thrombocytopaenia
Neurological	Headaches, confusion, tremor, visual and sensory disturbances, neuromuscular weakness, coma
Renal	Nocturia, polyuria, thirst, renal osteodystrophy
Skin	Pruritus, pigmentation, bruising, infections

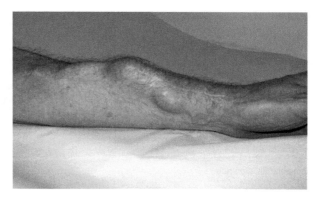

Figure 3.19 A surgically created arteriovenous fistula

Patients should avoid wearing tight clothing or a wristwatch on the fistula arm. They should check the fistula every day (by palpation) and never allow blood samples or blood pressure to be taken from that arm.

Diagnosis

Chronic kidney disease is diagnosed by:

- Clinical history and presentation
- Rising plasma urea and creatinine levels and a falling glomerular filtration rate (GFR). An estimate can be provided by the laboratory (eGFR) from serum creatinine, gender, age and race (MDRD4v equation).

Investigations as dictated by the nature of clinical disease.

Management

Management of CKD is particularly aimed at reducing cardiovascular risk, the main cause of mortality. Reversible causes of CKD should be treated, such as infection and urinary tract obstruction. Nephrotoxic drugs should also be avoided.

Management aims to:

- Modify lifestyle: smoking cessation, weight reduction, regular exercise and dietary salt restriction
- Lower blood pressure: ACE (angiotensin converting enzyme) inhibitor or ARB (angiotensin receptor blockers)
- Lower cardiovascular risk: lipid lowering therapy and low dose aspirin
- Correct anaemia: erythropoiesis stimulating agents (ESA) may be required. Recombinant erythropoietin is administered regularly if the haemoglobin level is <8.5g/dL and is needed in approximately 75% of patients in late CKD.

Also involved are:

- Medicines management: all patients with CKD should avoid potential nephrotoxic agents (in particular NSAIDs) or other metabolic complications (e.g. hyperkalaemia or metabolic acidosis)
- Bone management: calcium carbonate, vitamin D3 or its synthetic analogue, a low phosphate diet and a bisphosphonate may be needed for the management of renal osteodystrophy. Parathyroidectomy is occasionally indicated in resistant cases
- Dialysis: this removes waste metabolites and restores normal plasma biochemistry and becomes essential in ESRF. It includes:
  - Peritoneal dialysis: continuous ambulatory peritoneal dialysis (CAPD) and intermittent peritoneal dialysis involve placement of a catheter into the abdominal peritoneal cavity. Several litres of dialysate are exchanged throughout the day
  - Haemodialysis: carried out either at home or as an outpatient, for two or three, 3–6 hourly sessions per week. An arteriovenous fistula or an indwelling tunnelled cuffed catheter is usually created to facilitate infusions. The patient is heparinised during dialysis to keep both the infusion lines and the dialysis machine tubing patent. Infection control to prevent cross-infection of hepatitis viruses, HIV and other blood-borne agents is of paramount importance
  - Haemofiltration: renal replacement therapy (RRT) may be in the form of dialysis, but this requires massive fluid shifts, which are inappropriate for critically ill patients. Filtration is a slower method, which is less stressful for the cardiovascular system. This process uses a highly permeable membrane and allows removal of plasma water and waste metabolites. It is indicated for only a small number of patients with ESRF, generally in the intensive care setting. Continuous venous–venous haemofiltration (CVVHF) is the preferred form of RRT and allows for slow adjustments of fluid balance
- Renal transplantation may become necessary in ESRF and offers the potential for complete rehabilitation without the need for regular dialysis. The transplanted kidney is usually sited in the right iliac fossa of the abdomen and patients require long-term immunosuppressive therapy with drugs such as corticosteroids, azathioprine, ciclosporin, tacrolimus and mycophenolate. Complications of renal transplantation include:
  - Rejection of the transplanted kidney
  - Increased risk of atheroma and ischaemic heart disease
  - Ciclosporin-induced nephropathy and gingival swelling
  - Recurrent infection secondary to immunosuppression
  - Malignancy secondary to immunosuppression, including lip and mouth cancer.

Oral health care relevance

- The impact on the dental management of the patient in CKD depends on the stage of the disease, whether the patient is undergoing dialysis, as well as co-morbidities such as hypertension, diabetes mellitus and anaemia.

- The main considerations include:
  - Haemorrhage: effective haemostasis must be assured following invasive dental procedures and full local haemostatic measures instigated. If the patient is undergoing haemodialysis, dental treatment should be provided the day after dialysis once the effects of heparin have worn off
  - Infection: this can have serious consequences. Dental sepsis should be managed without delay, patients being asked to contact the dentist immediately if they believe they may be developing a dental infection. Due regard must be given to the nature of the antibiotics used, as detailed below
  - Drug therapy: in general this should ideally be minimised. Drugs excreted by the kidney may show exaggerated pharmacological effects and dosage reduction may be necessary. Non-steroidal anti-inflammatory drugs including aspirin are best avoided, but paracetamol can be safely used for analgesia. Antibiotics such as phenoxymethylpenicillin, amoxicillin and erythromycin can be used safely although their dose may need to be reduced in severe disease. Tetracyclines are best avoided, with the possible exception of doxycycline. It is sensible to discuss the proposed treatment with the renal physician concerned, prior to prescribing. Lidocaine can be used as normal in patients with chronic renal failure
  - If the patient is receiving a bisphosphonate, the potential for osteochemonecrosis (Figure 3.20) must be considered and appropriate measures should be taken to minimise this complication.

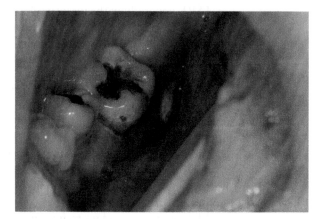

Figure 3.20   Osteochemonecrosis

Orofacial manifestations in CKD include xerostomia, dysgeusia, features relating to anaemia, osteoporosis with loss of lamina dura, giant cell lesions (brown tumours) due to secondary hyperparathyroidism, mucosal purpura and, in severe cases, erythemopultaceous stomatitis.

Thyrotoxicosis

Hyperthyroidism is associated:

- usually: with a diffuse goitre due to autoimmune Graves disease (primary hyperthyroidism) when there are thyroid-stimulating autoantibodies against thyroid TSH receptor (TRAbs) and microsomal antibodies (TMAbs)
- sometimes: with a hyperfunctioning (toxic) nodular goitre (thyroid adenomas) producing excess thyroxine
- rarely: with thyroiditis, thyroid overdosage or ectopic thyroid tissue.

Clinical features

Hyperthyroidism mimics adrenaline (epinephrine) effects, and can cause:

- Anxiety
- Tremor
- Sweating and heat intolerance
- Tachycardia, arrhythmias or cardiac failure
- Anorexia
- Vomiting
- Diarrhoea
- Weight loss.

Clinical signs

Exophthalmos (Figure 3.21), eyelid lag and eyelid retraction may be seen.

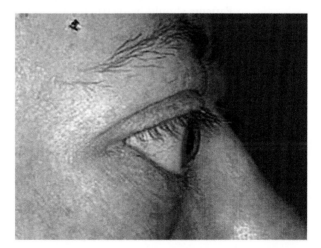

Figure 3.21   Exophthalmos

Exophthalmos refers to the abnormal protrusion of an eye from the orbit. Any swelling within the unyielding bony walls of the orbit will push the eyeball forwards and present as an exophthalmos. Bilateral exophthalmos is typical of Graves disease, a type of autoimmune hyperthyroidism.

Diagnosis

The diagnosis should be confirmed by:

- Raised serum levels of thyroid hormones (T3 and T4)
- Circulating auto-antibodies (TMAbs and TRAbs)
- Radioactive iodine uptake test or thyroid scan.

Management

- Carbimazole: the usual anti-thyroid drug but it can suppress the bone marrow and can cause rashes or mouth ulcers
- ^{131}Iodine: can result in hypothyroidism or hyposalivation
- Surgery: effective, but leads to hypothyroidism in about 30% of patients
- Beta-blockers: achieve rapid control of cardiac complications.

Oral health care relevance

- In uncontrolled hyperthyroidism, patients are tense and anxious.
- Benzodiazepines may potentiate anti-thyroid drugs, and therefore nitrous oxide, which is more rapidly controllable, is probably safer for conscious sedation.
- Anti-thyroid drugs such as carbimazole occasionally cause agranulocytosis, which in turn may predispose patients to oral and pharyngeal ulceration. Patients should be instructed to stop the medication if they develop a sore throat and contact their doctor for a full blood count.

Cushing disease and Cushing syndrome

- Cushing disease is due to sustained overproduction of cortisol in adrenal hyperplasia secondary to excess adrenocorticotrophic hormone (ACTH) production by pituitary adenomas.
- Cushing syndrome is similar but caused by increased corticosteroid levels of any other aetiology (including exogenously administered steroids).

Clinical features

The most obvious features are:

- Truncal obesity, affecting face (moon face), interscapular region (buffalo hump) and trunk, but sparing limbs
- Hypertension
- Hyperglycaemia and diabetes mellitus
- Osteoporosis, muscle weakness, purpura, skin thinning and striae
- Hirsutism and acne
- Oligomenorrhoea
- Infections
- Psychoses.

Clinical signs

A 'moon face' is characteristic of Cushing disease/syndrome (Figure 3.22). Other physical signs include truncal obesity, a buffalo hump and sometimes muscle wasting of the limbs, acne, atrophic skin with bruising and striae, and hirsutism.

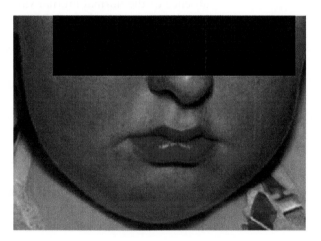

Figure 3.22 Moon face

Buffalo hump (Figure 3.23) is an accumulation of fat on the back of the neck and upper back. Common causes include Cushing disease, extended use of some steroids (glucocorticoids such as prednisone, cortisone and hydrocortisone) or extreme obesity. Buffalo hump is an unusual adverse effect of anti-retroviral treatment with protease inhibitors for HIV/AIDS.

Diagnosis

- Facial photographs from the past and more recently, may show the development of a moon face.

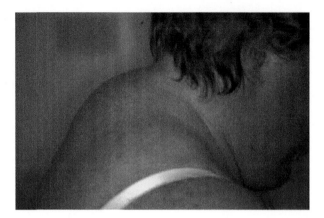

Figure 3.23   Buffalo hump

- Cushing disease is confirmed by:
  - raised plasma cortisol levels
  - absence of the normal diurnal variation in plasma cortisol
  - low dose overnight dexamethasone suppression test.
- Localisation of the cause relies on:
  - Corticotrophin-releasing hormone (CRH) stimulation test
  - Levels of ACTH
  - Pituitary MRI, tomography, abdominal CT and adrenal ultrasound.

Management

- In Cushing disease, the pituitary tumour is treated by trans-sphenoidal microadenectomy.
- In Cushing syndrome if due to localised adrenal disease, the responsible adrenal gland is usually irradiated or excised.
- Corticosteroid replacement is subsequently necessary.

Oral health care relevance

- The possibility of adrenocortical crisis must be considered and corticosteroid cover may be required prior to surgical interventions.
- Diabetes mellitus and hypertension are features of Cushing disease/syndrome and precautions appropriate to these conditions should be taken.

Addison disease

- Caused by autoantibodies to the adrenal cortex, there is atrophy and failure of cortisol (hydrocortisone) and aldosterone secretion.

- Hypoadrenocorticism is occasionally secondary to tuberculosis, histoplasmosis, malignancy, haemorrhage, sarcoidosis, amyloidosis or adrenalectomy.

Clinical features

- Low cortisol:
  - Predisposes to hypotension and hypoglycaemia
  - Stimulates the hypothalamopituitary axis causing release of pro-opiomelanocortin, which has ACTH and melanocyte stimulating hormone (MSH) activity and can cause hyperpigmentation.
- Low aldosterone:
  - Causes low sodium, reduced fluid volume and hypotension.
- Patients with hypoadrenocorticism can thus suffer from:
  - Anorexia, nausea, vomiting and diarrhoea
  - Fatigue and weakness
  - Lethargy
  - Dizziness and postural hypotension
  - Weight loss
  - Hyperpigmentation.
- The lack of adrenocortical reserve means patients are vulnerable to stress such as infection, trauma, surgery or anaesthesia, which can cause an acute adrenal (Addisonian) crisis, characterised by collapse, bradycardia, hypotension, profound weakness, hypoglycaemia, vomiting and dehydration.

Clinical signs

In Addison disease, the low serum cortisol levels stimulate increased production of ACTH from the anterior pituitary gland, resulting in increased skin pigmentation, especially within creases (Figure 3.24a), areas of mild trauma and mucosal and gingival pigmentation (Figure 3.24b).

Vitiligo (Figure 3.25), caused by an autoimmune destruction of melanocytes within the skin, is often seen in isolation but may be seen in other organ-specific autoimmune conditions such as type 1 diabetes, thyroid disorders and pernicious anaemia.

Diagnosis

Diagnosis of Addison disease is confirmed by:

- Hypotension
- Low plasma cortisol levels
- Depressed cortisol responses to tetracosactide (Synacthen – synthetic ACTH) stimulation

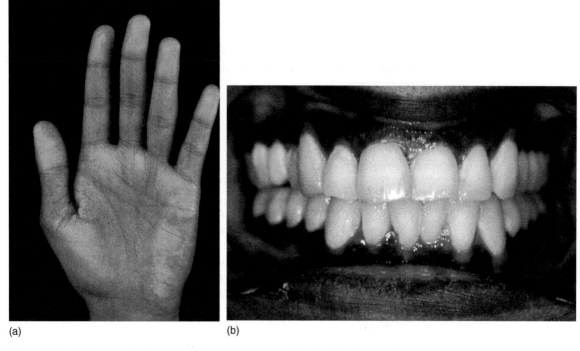

(a)   (b)

Figure 3.24   (a) Increased skin pigmentation in creases and (b) gingival pigmentation

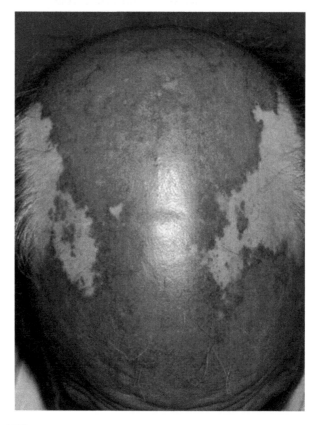

Figure 3.25   Vitiligo

- ACTH levels; raised in primary but low or normal in secondary hypoadrenocorticism
- Plasma electrolyte assays: sodium may be low and potassium raised
- Plasma glucose assay: hypoglycaemia is common
- Serum autoantibodies
- Radiography, CT or MRI scans of skull, chest and abdomen.

Management

- Oral hydrocortisone and fludrocortisone acetate.

Oral health care relevance

- The risk of precipitating hypotensive collapse is such that corticosteroids must be given prior to invasive dental treatment. Such patients may be best managed within a hospital setting.
- Hyperpigmented mucosae, including the gingivae (Figure 3.24b), are seen in more than 75% of patients.
- The dental team must be familiar with the emergency management of adrenocortical insufficiency.

4 Gastrointestinal conditions

Peptic ulcer disease

An ulcer is a break in the continuity of an epithelial surface that exposes the underlying connective tissue. Peptic ulcer disease (PUD) develops in, or close to, acid-secreting areas in the stomach (gastric ulcer) or proximal duodenum (duodenal ulcer). Peptic ulcer disease affects up to 15% of the general population, mostly men over the age of 45 years.

Helicobacter pylori (a spiral bacterium) infection is a key factor in the development of 70–90% of PUD. Possible damaging actions of *H. pylori* include:

- Increased gastric acid secretion
- Loss of the mucus protective layer
- Increased secretion of pepsinogen
- Urease production, which converts urea into bicarbonate and ammonia (both strong bases) and is the basis for diagnosis of *H. pylori* by the 'breath test'.

Peptic ulcer disease is also occasionally associated with:

- Raised gastrin levels as in Zollinger-Ellison syndrome (a gastrin-producing tumour), hyperparathyroidism and chronic renal failure
- Drugs (non-steroidal anti-inflammatory drugs [NSAIDs], corticosteroids, smoking, alcohol)
- Stress.

Clinical features

The main feature of PUD is epigastric pain, often relieved by antacids but many patients are symptomless or suffer from only occasional dyspepsia. Complications include haemorrhage, perforation and pyloric obstruction (stenosis).

Clinical signs

An endoscopic view of peptic ulceration is shown in Figure 4.1.

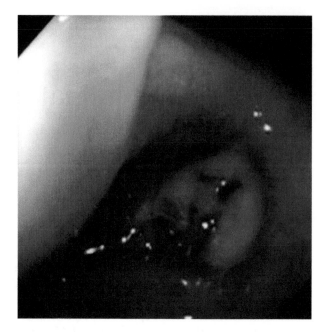

Figure 4.1   Peptic ulceration

Diagnosis

Patients less than 45 years old who present with typical ulcer symptoms should be screened for *H. pylori* via a breath test or serologically. Older individuals require an upper gastrointestinal endoscopy, and multiple gastric biopsies are taken to exclude the presence of malignancy should an ulcer be present. Biopsy specimens are also tested for the presence of *H. pylori*. Studies of gastric acid or serum gastrin levels may be helpful and, if gastric outlet obstruction is suspected, a barium meal may be diagnostically helpful.

Management

Management of PUD involves conservative measures:

- Dietary modification (frequent small meals with no fried foods)
- Smoking cessation
- Alcohol moderation.

H. pylori-positive individuals should be given 'triple therapy' normally consisting of 7 days:

- Amoxicillin plus
- Clarithromycin plus
- A proton-pump inhibitor (e.g. omeprazole or lansoprazole).

Drugs that block histamine (H2) receptors such as cimetidine and ranitidine may be used to reduce gastric acid secretion. Prostaglandin analogues such as misoprostol promote healing and are indicated in patients with PUD from whom NSAIDs cannot be withdrawn.

Surgical interventions are reserved for those with complications. Gastric ulcers may be managed by antrectomy with gastroduodenal anastomosis or partial gastrectomy; duodenal ulcers are managed rarely with vagotomy and pyloroplasty.

Oral health care relevance

- Antacids can interfere with the absorption of various anti-microbials, particularly tetracyclines, which become chelated (bound and thus less effective).
- Chronic blood loss from PUD may result in iron deficiency (with or without anaemia), leading to aphthous stomatitis, glossitis and candidosis including angular cheilitis.
- *Helicobacter pylori* can be found in saliva but there is no reliable evidence that it causes mouth ulcers or malodour.
- Proton pump inhibitors may produce xerostomia. Omeprazole may also provoke erythema multiforme and loss of taste.

Stomach (gastric) cancer

The stomach is a frequent site of cancer, usually adenocarcinoma. Men are affected nearly twice as often as women. The aetiology is obscure but risk factors include:

- Genetic influences: common in Japanese and where there is a positive history in first degree relatives; people who carry mutations of the breast cancer genes *BRCA1* and *BRCA2* may also have a higher rate
- Male gender
- Older age
- Smoking
- Occupations: workers in coal, metal and rubber industries
- Atrophic gastritis
- Achlorhydria
- *Helicobacter pylori*
- Diet (smoked foods, salted fish and meat, and pickled vegetables)
- Pernicious anaemia
- Blood group A
- Obesity.

Clinical features

Early symptoms of stomach cancer may closely mimic PUD. Indigestion, upper abdominal pain, anorexia, weight loss, anaemia, nausea, vomiting, haematemesis (vomiting blood) or melaena (stools black and tarry with blood) may develop. Later there can be intestinal obstruction causing vomiting, or bile duct obstruction causing jaundice.

Metastases are mainly to liver, peritoneum (causing ascites), lungs, bones or brain.

Clinical signs

Gastric carcinoma can metastasise widely, occasionally to the skin (Figure 4.2).

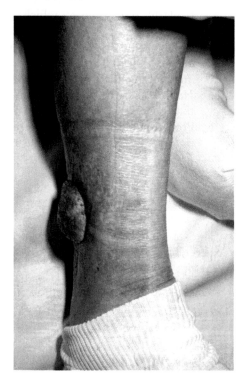

Figure 4.2   Metastasis from gastric carcinoma

Diagnosis

The diagnosis is usually confirmed by gastroscopy and biopsy and barium imaging.

Management

Surgery is the main treatment but often only palliative. There is about a 15% 5-year survival rate.

Oral health care relevance

Oral effects of anaemia (glossitis, ulcers, angular stomatitis) can be an initial sign. Iron deficiency in a male usually results from chronic haemorrhage, often from the gastrointestinal tract, e.g. stomach, large bowel neoplasm or ulceration.

Paraneoplastic pemphigus, whilst more typically associated with lymphoreticular malignancies, may also be a sign of underlying gastric carcinoma.

Orofacial metastases from gastric carcinoma are uncommon, usually in the mandible and may cause swelling, pain, paraesthesia, loosening of teeth or sockets that fail to heal. Metastases may be first detected in a lower cervical (supraclavicular) lymph node, usually on the left side (Troisier sign).

Inflammatory bowel disease

Inflammatory bowel disease (IBD) is a collective term that encompasses the spectrum of disease seen in Crohn disease and ulcerative colitis (UC). A comparison of Crohn disease with UC is outlined in Table 4.1.

Table 4.1   Comparison of Crohn disease and ulcerative colitis

Features	Crohn disease	Ulcerative colitis
Main site affected	Ileum	Colorectum
Other sites affected	Any part of the gastrointestinal tract, including the mouth	Terminal ileum
Pathology	Transmural granulomatous inflammation	Superficial inflammation
Abdominal pain	Prominent	Less prominent
Bloody diarrhoea	Common	Prominent
Fistulae and abscesses	Possible	Rare
Colonic carcinoma risk	Low	High
Iron deficiency	Common	Common
Folate deficiency	Common	Uncommon
Other deficiencies	Vitamin B12 deficiency common	Rare

Crohn disease is a chronic inflammatory disease of unknown cause, seen mainly in Caucasians and with a bimodal age distribution of disease onset with peaks at 20 and 50 years. Current evidence suggests it may represent an abnormal mucosal T-lymphocyte response to commensal bacteria in genetically predisposed individuals. Microscopically, there is submucosal chronic non-caseating granulomatous inflammation characterised by multinucleate giant cells. The inflammatory response is mediated by factors such as tumour necrosis factor alpha. Implicated are the *CARD15* gene and perhaps infection with *Mycobacterium paratuberculosis*.

Ulcerative colitis is an inflammatory bowel disease that most often affects people between the ages of 15 and 40 years. The aetiology is unknown but both genetic and environmental factors contribute. HLA Class II alleles, interleukin-1 and the multi-drug resistance *MDR1* genes have been implicated, and there is a relationship with an increased number of adherent *Bacteroides* spp. and *Enterobacteriaceae* spp. in inflamed bowel segments. Conversely, cigarette smoking and appendectomy have both been shown to protect against ulcerative colitis. Inflammation and ulceration of the superficial layers of the mucosa are followed by pseudopolyp formation.

Clinical features

Crohn disease can affect any part of the gastrointestinal tract but predominantly affects the ileocaecal region, typically with ulceration, fissuring and fibrosis. It may cause abdominal pain mimicking appendicitis and usually presents with an alteration of bowel habit as well as features of malabsorption. Diarrhoea, bleeding and painful defaecation are typical.

Ulcerative colitis can affect any part or the whole of the large intestine, but frequently affects the lower colon and rectum. Typical features are diarrhoea with stools containing intermixed mucus, blood and pus. In severe cases, abdominal pain, fever, anorexia and weight loss predominate.

Complications of IBD include weight loss, anaemia, gastrointestinal obstruction and, particularly in Crohn disease, perianal fissures, fistulae and abscess formation. Non-gastrointestinal features include: conjunctivitis, uveitis, iritis, finger clubbing sacroileitis, skin disease (erythema nodosum and pyoderma gangrenosum), liver disease (primary sclerosing cholangitis), gallstones and renal calculi.

Patients with Crohn disease are at an increased risk of cancer but less so than those with UC. Individuals with poorly controlled UC for longer than 10 years' duration have a significantly increased risk of colorectal carcinoma. Disease extension through the muscular layers in UC may result in life-threatening toxic megacolon (the colon dilates and can perforate).

Clinical signs

Cutaneous manifestations can include fistula (Figure 4.3), pyoderma gangrenosum (see Figure 4.9) and other skin disorders (Figure 4.4), perianal tags and fissures (Figure 4.5).

Swelling of the face or lips may be seen (Figure 4.6).

The oral mucosa may appear cobblestoned (Figure 4.7); oral mucosal tagging, ulceration, angular cheilitis (see Figure 5.1) and linear or hyperplastic gingivitis may be signs of Crohn disease.

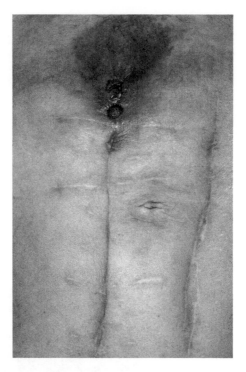

Figure 4.3 A fistula in Crohn disease following on from previous surgery

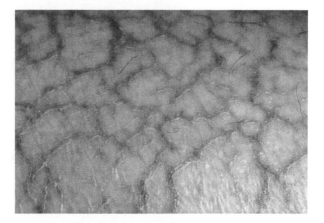

Figure 4.4 The skin in a patient with malabsorption

Leukonychia (white nails; Figure 4.8) are typically seen in chronic low albumin states such as inflammatory bowel disease, chronic renal disease (albumin loss) or chronic liver disease (reduced albumin synthesis). Other listed causes are heart disease and arsenic poisoning. The fingernails are predominantly white, although the distal areas remain normal.

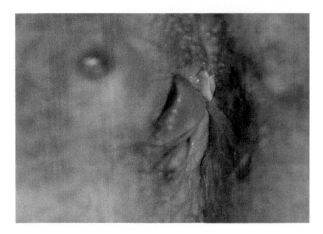

Figure 4.5   Perianal tags seen in Crohn disease

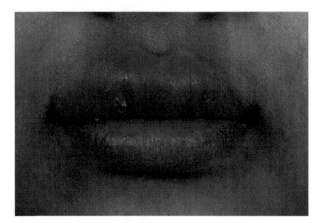

Figure 4.6   Swollen lips in Crohn disease

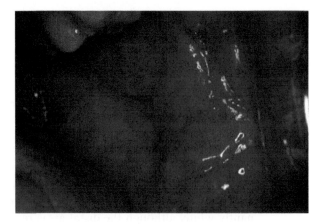

Figure 4.7   Cobblestoned appearance of oral mucosa in Crohn disease

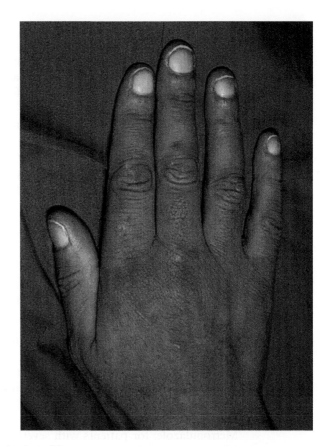

Figure 4.8   Leukonychia

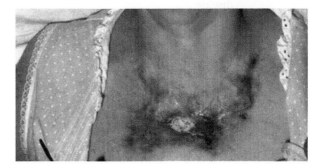

Figure 4.9   Pyoderma gangrenosum

Cutaneous necrotic lesions may be seen in UC (pyoderma gangrenosum; Figure 4.9).

Diagnosis

There are no specific diagnostic tests for either Crohn disease or UC. Investigations include:

- Blood count: anaemia is common and varies depending on whether iron, folate or vitamin B12 are deficient
- Erythrocyte sedimentation rate (ESR): a non-specific blood marker of inflammation, which is usually raised, as is the C-reactive protein (CRP)
- Plain-film radiography: should be performed in severe colitis to exclude toxic dilatation of the colon
- Contrast radiography (barium studies): may demonstrate an altered mucosal pattern
- Ultrasound and computed tomography (CT): may delineate abscesses
- Endoscopy (sigmoidoscopy, colonoscopy) and mucosal biopsy: invariably demonstrate non-caseating granulomatous disease in Crohn disease, but non-specific inflammation with goblet cell depletion and crypt abscesses in UC.

Management

Medical therapy includes conservative measures (nutritional support) and drug therapy:

- 5-Aminosalicylates (mesalazine, olsalazine): induce and maintain remission in mild UC and colonic Crohn disease
- Corticosteroids may be given orally, intravenously or topically in the form of steroid enemas: exert multiple anti-inflammatory effects
- Azathioprine and mercaptopurine: for patients unresponsive to aminosalicylates
- Metronidazole: for patients with severe perianal Crohn disease
- Methotrexate and ciclosporin: used occasionally in patients with resistant disease
- Anti-tumour necrosis factor-alpha (TNF-α) antibodies (infliximab): for individuals with severe steroid-resistant Crohn disease.

Surgery in IBD is indicated for:

- Failure of medical therapy
- Treating complications from longstanding disease.

In Crohn disease recurrence is likely and fistulae often complicate surgery, therefore bowel resections are conservative and avoided if possible. The surgical options in UC depend on the extent of disease but generally consist of excision of diseased bowel with either re-anastomosis or ileostomy construction.

Oral health care relevance

- Crohn disease rarely complicates the dental management of the patient. Some patients may be treated with corticosteroids and appropriate considerations will apply.
- Broad spectrum antibiotics should be avoided where possible to minimise the risk of further gastrointestinal tract upset.

- Orofacial manifestations may include:
  - Orofacial granulomatosis: swelling of the face, lips and/or areas of the oral mucosa that may appear cobblestoned, oral mucosal tagging, ulceration, angular cheilitis and linear or hyperplastic gingivitis
  - Aphthous-like ulceration: this may be a primary phenomenon due to active Crohn disease or secondary to the haematinic deficiency that may result from the condition (in particular, serum B12, if the condition is longstanding, and additionally iron and/or folate deficiencies).

Coeliac disease (gluten-sensitive enteropathy)

Coeliac disease, the most common genetic disease in Europe, is an autoimmune disorder in which there is hypersensitivity or toxic reaction of the small intestine mucosa to the gliadin component of gluten, a group of proteins found in all wheats, related grains (rye and barley) and possibly oats. Ingestion of gluten causes destruction of jejunal villi (villous atrophy) and inflammation, leading to malabsorption.

Coeliac disease may be associated with other autoimmune disorders (including Sjögren syndrome).

Clinical features

Coeliac disease may present at any age and mimic a variety of medical conditions. Although affected individuals may be asymptomatic or complain of lethargy and low grade malaise, coeliac disease can result in malabsorption leading to growth retardation, abdominal pain, steatorrhoea and behavioural changes. Vitamin and mineral deficiencies may result in anaemia, osteomalacia, bleeding tendencies and neurological disorders.

Intestinal lymphomas arise in about 6% of individuals.

Clinical signs

Coeliac disease may present with diarrhoea, steatorrhoea, abdominal discomfort, weight loss, mouth ulcers and anaemia. Rare complications are tetany, osteomalacia, neurological symptoms and lymphoma.

Dermatitis herpetiformis (Figure 4.10) is an extremely itchy rash, which is typically symmetrically distributed mainly over the elbows, knees, shoulders, buttocks and scalp. Because of the itching, it is unusual to see vesicles as these are burst by scratching. Most patients have a gluten-sensitive enteropathy (coeliac disease) although this is usually asymptomatic. Dapsone will usually control the rash within hours and on stopping the drug symptoms rapidly recur. A gluten-free diet will improve the gastrointestinal lesions and also improve the skin lesions.

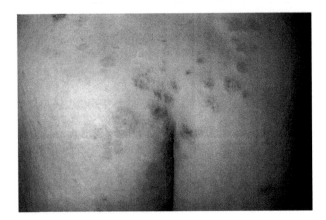

Figure 4.10   Dermatitis herpetiformis

Diagnosis

As the clinical features of coeliac disease are usually non-specific, investigations are needed to establish the diagnosis. These include:

- Full blood count: anaemia is present in 50% of patients
- Haematinics: ferritin and folate levels may be low secondary to malabsorption. Serum B12 deficiency is rare
- Serum antibody screening: antibodies (IgA isotype) to endomysium (the connective tissue stroma covering individual muscle fibres) and tissue transglutaminase have high specificity and sensitivity for coeliac disease and have replaced tests for anti-gliadin and anti-reticulin antibodies
- Endoscopic biopsy of jejunal mucosa: shows villous atrophy. The biopsy, if positive, is repeated after a gluten-free diet has been maintained for 3 months.

Management

It is important to diagnose coeliac disease and to institute a gluten-free diet, even in those with minimal symptoms, as early as possible in order to prevent long-term complications (intestinal lymphoma).

Treatment includes correction of nutritional deficiencies, and a gluten-free diet for life. Instead of wheat flour, patients can use potato, rice, soy or bean flour and can buy gluten-free bread, pasta and other products. Plain meat, fish, fruits and vegetables do not contain gluten.

Patients require continued supervision, as it is often difficult to comply with such a diet, especially if eating away from home.

Oral health care relevance

- Patients with untreated coeliac disease may present with aphthous–like ulcers.

- As a consequence of folate and/or iron deficiency (with or without anaemia) these patients may also have candidosis or glossitis (see Figures 5.1 and 5.2).
- Rarely, patients may develop oral manifestations of dermatitis herpetiformis.
- There is an association between Sjögren syndrome and coeliac disease.

Colon cancer (colorectal cancer)

Colon cancer is the third most common cancer in the UK and usually arises in the rectum or pelvic (sigmoid) colon. Men are affected almost twice as frequently as women. Risk factors include:

- Heredity: familial polyposis coli
- Inflammatory bowel disease, especially ulcerative colitis
- Smoking
- Diet high in red meat and fat and low in fibre, fruit and vegetables
- Cholecystectomy.

Clinical features

Abdominal pain, change in bowel habit, melaena, weight loss, anaemia, intestinal obstruction or perforation may occur.

Clinical signs

Metastases can be widespread, especially involving the liver (Figure 4.11).

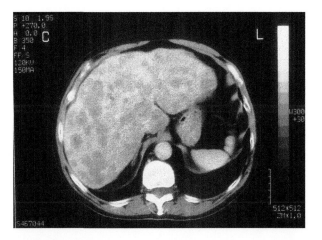

Figure 4.11   Metastases to the liver

Diagnosis

Faecal occult blood (FOB), ultrasound, CT, barium enema, sigmoidoscopy, colonoscopy and magnetic resonance imaging (MRI) may be required.

Management

Surgical resection is the usual treatment. The overall 5-year survival rate is about 50%. Radiotherapy may be useful for dealing with pain from recurrences. Chemotherapy (capecitabine, irinotecan hydrochloride, oxaliplatin, raltitrexed) may be used in advanced colorectal carcinoma. Metastatic carcinoma may be treated with bevacizumab and cetuximab.

Serial monitoring for carcinoembryonic antigen (CEA) may help detect recurrences.

Oral health care relevance

Multiple mandibular osteomas may be markers of an enhanced risk of colorectal cancer as a consequence of Gardner syndrome (familial polyposis coli together with extracolonic tumours – osteomas of the jaws and skull, thyroid cancer, fibromas, and epidermoid and sebaceous cysts).

5

Haematological conditions

Anaemia

Anaemia is defined as a haemoglobin (Hb) level below the normal for the age, gender and ethnic background of the individual (female <11 g/dL; male <13 g/dL). Its causes are outlined in Table 5.1. Most common is iron deficiency anaemia from chronic blood loss. Deficiency anaemias may also be caused by folate or vitamin B12 deficiency.

Table 5.1 Causes of anaemia

Nature of anaemia	Cause
Increased RBC loss	Menstrual blood loss
	Gastrointestinal blood loss
	Haemolysis
Reduced RBC production	Haematinic deficiency
	Bone marrow infiltration
	Aplastic anaemia
Increased tissue requirements	Puberty
	Pregnancy
Decreased tissue requirements	Hypothyroidism

RBC, red blood cell.

Excessive red blood cell (RBC) breakdown in haemolytic anaemias, especially sickle cell disease, are relevant especially when general anaesthesia is considered, since the erythrocytes lyse if there is hypoxia.

Anaemia may also be classified on the basis of RBC size (Table 5.2).

Clinical features

Patients are commonly symptomless if the onset of anaemia is slow. However, as the anaemia worsens and the oxygen carrying capacity of the blood falls, cardiac symptoms and signs develop (dyspnoea, palpitations, tachycardia, flow murmurs and ultimately cardiac failure). Pallor of the oral mucosa, conjunctiva or palmar creases suggests severe anaemia, but skin colour can be misleading.

Table 5.2 Classification of anaemias according to RBC size

Mean cell volume (MCV)	Cause
Microcytic (Low MCV, <76 fL)	Iron deficiency Haemoglobinopathy
Normocytic (Normal MCV, 76–96 fL)	Acute haemorrhage Haemolysis Anaemia of chronic disease Malignancy Bone marrow failure
Macrocytic (High MCV, >96 fL)	Vitamin B12 deficiency Folate deficiency Alcohol Liver disease Hypothyroidism

Anaemia may worsen pre-existing coronary, peripheral and cerebrovascular disease.

Clinical signs

Angular stomatitis, glossitis and koilonychia (nails that have lost their natural convex curvature, becoming flat or even concave [spoon-shaped nails]) are usually signs of chronic iron deficiency anaemia (Figure 5.1). Oral candidosis, aphthous ulceration and, in severe chronic cases, dysphagia or post-cricoid web may occur.

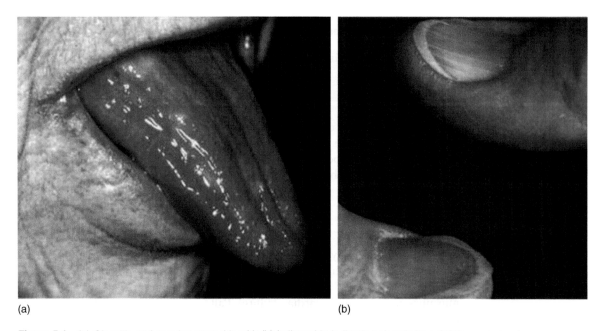

(a)   (b)

Figure 5.1 (a) Glossitis and angular stomatitis with (b) koilonychia indicating chronic iron deficiency anaemia

Pernicious anaemia, a type of megaloblastic anaemia caused by an inability to absorb vitamin B12 due to a lack of intrinsic factor in gastric secretions, may present with sore tongue and glossitis (Figure 5.2), mouth ulcers or angular stomatitis. The most common causes of megaloblastic anaemia are vitamin B12 and folic acid deficiency; rare causes include leukaemia, myelofibrosis, multiple myeloma, Rogers syndrome (an autosomal recessive thiamine-responsive anaemia, with diabetes mellitus and sensorineural deafness), Imerslund–Grasbeck syndrome (an autosomal recessive B12-responsive anaemia), drugs – chemotherapy that affects DNA synthesis (e.g. methotrexate), alcohol or phenytoin and, in children, coeliac disease and chronic infectious enteritis. Subacute combined degeneration of the spinal cord is a potential complication of longstanding vitamin B12 deficiency, which results in various central and peripheral neurological disorders.

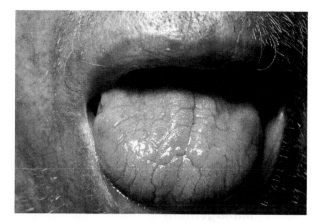

Figure 5.2 Glossitis in pernicious anaemia

Chronic haemorrhage is the most common cause of iron deficiency, usually from the uterus or gastrointestinal tract. The rare Osler–Weber–Rendu syndrome, or hereditary hemorrhagic telangiectasia (Figure 5.3), has a wide spectrum of presentations: patients may be asymptomatic or have multiple organ involvement, presenting at any age. The major cause of morbidity and mortality due to this disorder lies in the multiorgan arteriovenous malformations (AVMs) and their associated haemorrhage that may lead to severe iron deficiency anaemia. More than 20% of patients with Osler–Weber–Rendu syndrome have AVMs, and it is therefore recommended that they receive antibiotic prophylaxis prior to dental and surgical interventions to reduce embolic abscesses (e.g. brain abscesses).

Diagnosis

Anaemia is diagnosed from the Hb level but the precise nature and underlying cause must be established. Depending on the clinical presentation the following investigations may be indicated:

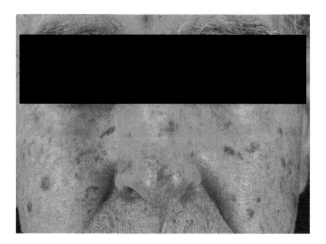

Figure 5.3   Telangiectasia of Osler–Weber–Rendu syndrome

- Full blood count: to ascertain Hb level and RBC indices
- Blood film: may demonstrate abnormal RBC forms (sickle cells in sickle cell disease and pencil cells in iron deficiency anaemia)
- Haemoglobin electrophoresis: haemoglobinopathy screening
- Haematinics: serum vitamin B12, folate and ferritin levels
- Endoscopy: to identify sources of gastrointestinal blood loss
- Bone marrow biopsy: to exclude bone marrow infiltration and disease.

Management

The key to anaemia management is the establishment and treatment of the underlying cause. Haematinic deficiency states must then be corrected with iron, folic acid and/or vitamin B12 supplements as appropriate.

Blood transfusion may be indicated if the onset of anaemia has been rapid so as to prevent worsening of ischaemic symptoms. In end-stage renal failure erythropoietin is administered regularly to encourage haemopoiesis.

Oral health care relevance

- Anaemia compromises the oxygen carrying capacity of the blood and this is a consideration in sedative techniques. Supplemental nasal oxygen would be a reasonable precaution in patients with mild anaemia. A haemoglobin of 9 g/dL or less classifies the patient as American Society of Anaesthesiologists (ASA) group III and precludes sedation within the primary care setting.
- Iron, folate and B12 deficiency anaemias may manifest orofacially as mouth ulcers, atrophic glossitis and candidosis, with angular stomatitis being seen particularly in iron deficiency anaemia.

Bleeding tendencies

Warfarin used as a prophylactic anticoagulant is the main cause of a bleeding tendency. Inherited blood coagulation factor defects, and platelet disorders are the other main causes.

Von Willebrand disease

Von Willebrand disease (vWD) is the most common inherited bleeding disorder: some subtypes are autosomal dominant conditions. It affects both males and females, and is due to a deficiency of von Willebrand factor (vWF).

Von Willebrand factor is synthesised in endothelium and megakaryocytes, mediates platelet adhesion to damaged endothelium and protects factor VIII from proteolytic degradation. A deficiency of vWF therefore results in defective platelet adhesion and reduced blood levels of factor VIII.

Clinical features

Von Willebrand disease may be classified as follows:

- Types 1 and 2: disease is mild and is characterised by bleeding from mucous membranes – nose bleeds, gingival haemorrhage and gastrointestinal blood loss. Excessive haemorrhage may occur after dental treatment and surgery
- Type 3: bleeding is more severe than in types 1 and 2 but joint and muscle bleeds characteristic of haemophilia are rare.

Clinical signs

- Bleeding from mucous membranes
- Excessive haemorrhage after dental treatment (Figure 5.4).

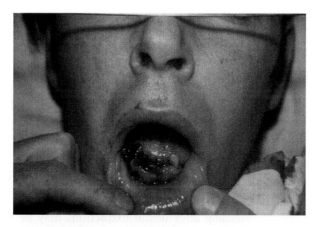

Figure 5.4   Haemorrhage following dental treatment in a patient with von Willebrand disease

Diagnosis

Von Willebrand disease is characterised by:

- Reduced von Willebrand factor levels
- Reduced factor VIII levels
- Reduced platelet aggregation in the presence of ristocetin
- Prolonged activated partial thromboplastin time (APTT)
- Prolonged bleeding time.

Management

Before surgery, to reduce the risk of haemorrhage, patients with von Willebrand disease need treatment, which may include the administration of:

- Factor VIII concentrate
- Synthetic vasopressin (desmopressin).

Oral health care relevance

See *Oral health care relevance* under *Haemophilias*, p. 83.

Haemophilias

Haemophilia A (classic haemophilia) and B (Christmas disease; named after the first patient described) are X-linked recessive hereditary disorders (affect males almost exclusively), characterised by deficiencies in blood clotting factors VIII and IX respectively.

Haemophilia B is much more common and affects approximately 1 in 500 males: haemophilia A affects approximately 1 in 5000 males.

Clinical features

Haemophilia is characterised by excessive bleeding, particularly after trauma and, sometimes, spontaneously. Haemorrhage appears to stop immediately after the injury (due to normal vascular and platelet haemostatic responses) but intractable oozing with rapid blood loss soon follows. Haemorrhage is dangerous either because of:

- Acute blood loss and/or
- Bleeding into tissues – particularly the retina, brain, larynx, pharynx, joints and muscles.

Bleeding after dental extractions may be the initial presenting feature of the disease.

The severity of bleeding in haemophilia A correlates with the level of Factor VIII:coagulant (VIII:C) activity and degree of trauma:

- Factor VIII activity less than 1% results in severe haemophilia with spontaneous bleeding and typically presents in childhood with bleeding into muscles or joints (haemarthroses), easy bruising and prolonged bleeding from minor injuries.
- Factor VIII activity of 1–5% causes moderate haemophilia.
- Factor VIII level above 5% causes mild disease but comparatively minor trauma may still lead to significant blood loss.
- Factor VIII level above 25% causes very mild haemophilia, in which the patient may remain undiagnosed and can generally lead a normal life.

Carriers of haemophilia rarely manifest a bleeding tendency clinically.

Clinical signs

- Bleeding into tissues e.g. retina (Figure 5.5), muscle (Figure 5.6)
- Bleeding after dental extraction.

Diagnosis

The diagnosis of haemophilia is based upon the clinical presentation, a positive family history, coagulation studies and clotting factor assays. The following findings are typical:

- Normal prothrombin time (PT)
- Normal bleeding time

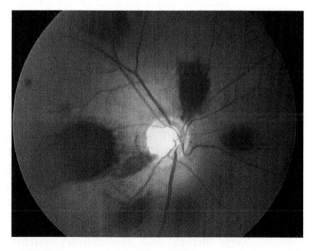

Figure 5.5   Retinal bleeding as a result of haemophilia

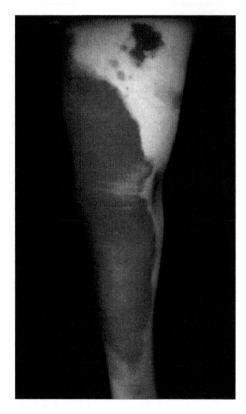

Figure 5.6   Widespread bleeding as a result of haemophilia

- Prolonged activated partial thromboplastin time
- Reduced factor VIII:C level (haemophilia A)
- Reduced factor IX level (haemophilia B)
- Normal levels of von Willebrand factor.

Management

People with haemophilia should be under the care of recognised Haemophilia Reference Centres.

- Factors VIII and IX must be replaced to adequate levels during episodes of bleeding and ascertained preoperatively. Recombinant products are now used: in the past, the use of blood or blood products led in some instances to infections with hepatitis viruses B and C, HIV, and prions.
- Synthetic vasopressin (desmopressin) acts to increase factor VIII levels and may be used in very mild haemophilia.

'Gene therapy' and 'gene-delivery systems' raise the possibility of a potential cure for haemophilia in the future.

Oral health care relevance

- Patients with these bleeding diatheses are generally managed in specialist units for invasive dental procedures where appropriate factor replacement therapy can be administered. Local haemostatic measures, including for example the use of oxidised cellulose gauze and topical tranexamic acid will also be implemented.
- Local anaesthesia is not contraindicated, but should be confined to local infiltration or periodontal ligament infiltration techniques. Regional anaesthesia must be avoided.
- Intravenous sedation can be undertaken but great care must be exercised to avoid unnecessary trauma during venous access.
- All dental interventions must be as atraumatic as possible. Even minor mucosal trauma, perhaps from a saliva ejector, can provoke troublesome bleeding or haematoma formation. This can be a very serious complication when there is floor of mouth or oropharyngeal involvement.
- Non-steroidal anti-inflammatory drugs (NSAIDs) including aspirin should be avoided.
- Orofacial manifestations include gingival bleeding and additionally mucosal purpura in von Willebrand disease.
- Patients who have received blood products have, in the past, been at risk of contracting infections (see above).

Leukaemias

Leukaemias are potentially lethal neoplastic disorders of bone marrow stem cells. The aetiology is unknown in most cases but may include a genetic predisposition and exposure to ionising radiation or chemicals such as benzene.

Leukaemias are classified by:

- Cell of origin (lymphoblast or non-lymphoblast)
- Cell maturity: immature (acute) versus mature (chronic).

The acute leukaemias account for nearly 50% of malignant disease in children and are characterised by primitive blast cells in the blood and bone marrow. Chronic leukaemias are predominantly diseases of late adult life and have a fairly benign course. Large numbers of mature leukocytes feature in the peripheral blood and bone marrow. This classification of leukaemias allows a patient's prognosis to be assessed and has implications for treatment.

Clinical features

The clinical features of leukaemia are variable but broadly reflect the degree of tissue infiltration by the leukaemic cells and the extent of bone marrow failure, which inevitably leads to loss of red cells (anaemia) and platelets (bleeding tendency) and, since the leukocytes are dysfunctional, also to infections (Table 5.3).

Table 5.3   Clinical features of leukaemia

Site of disease	Clinical manifestation
Bone marrow failure	
Anaemia	Pallor, lethargy, dyspnoea
Neutropaenia	Recurrent infection
Thrombocytopaenia	Mucosal bleeding and bruising
Tissue infiltration	
Lymphatics	Lymphadenopathy
Liver and spleen	Hepatosplenomegaly
Mediastinum	Hilar lymphadenopathy
Gingiva and skin	Gingival and skin deposits
Meninges and brain	Meningitis-like syndrome
Bone	Bone pain and pathological fractures

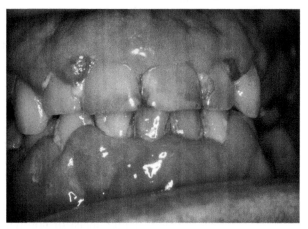

Figure 5.7   Gingival swelling and ulceration

Clinical signs

Lymph node enlargement is common, as is pallor and easy bruising. Gingival swelling, bleeding and ulceration may be seen (Figure 5.7). Some leukaemics present with persistent bleeding after tooth extraction.

Diagnosis

The diagnosis and prognosis of leukaemias are established by the following investigations:

- Haematological examination (full blood count and peripheral blood film)
- Bone marrow biopsy
- Cytochemistry and immunophenotyping for categorisation of cell type.

Supplementary investigations that may be required include:

- Lumbar puncture
- Chest radiography
- Computed tomography (CT)
- Magnetic resonance imaging (MRI).

Management

The treatment of leukaemia is dependent upon the accurate diagnosis and staging of the disease but generally involves combination chemotherapy with a variety of cytotoxic agents. Treatment consists of:

- Induction of remission and, increasingly, bone marrow transplantation
- Post-remission treatment (consolidation)
- Maintenance therapy.

Cytotoxic drugs damage all proliferating cells including epithelium, bone marrow and reproductive tissues and cause nausea and vomiting, impaired immunity, alopecia and mucositis.

Newer treatments include retinoids, monoclonal antibodies, peptide vaccines, T-cell infusions and cytokines such as granulocyte colony stimulating factor (GCSF).

Oral health care relevance

- The dental implications of the leukaemias are in part dependent on the nature and severity of the leukaemia, and the treatment. Acute leukaemias pose more dental management issues than do the chronic variants. In general, the major implications fall into the following broad areas:
  - Haemorrhage
  - Infection: particularly viral (e.g. herpes viruses) and fungal (e.g. candidoses)
  - Anaemia
  - Orofacial manifestations: related to the leukaemia or the therapy.
- Consultation with the patient's haematologist is mandatory in order to gain detailed information on the nature and level of risks involved, and indeed whether the patient is suitable, or not, for dental treatment in the primary care setting.
- Maintenance of a high level of oral hygiene is important to help reduce the risk of infection and is also important in minimising the need for invasive dental treatment with its attendant risks of bleeding and infection. Plaque control is important to minimise gingivitis, which is more likely to bleed.
- Amoxicillin (and ampicillin) may provoke skin rashes in leukaemic patients that are unrelated to penicillin hypersensitivity.
- Orofacial manifestations of leukaemias include:
  - Gingival swelling and haemorrhage as a consequence of leukaemic cell infiltration: seen in up to 30% of patients with acute myeloblastic leukaemia, but far less frequent in chronic leukaemias

- Mucosal purpura
- Mucosal pallor
- Fungal and viral infections
- Oral ulceration
- Lymphadenopathy
- Cytotoxic therapy can provoke oral ulceration and mucositis
- Busulfan can produce brown pigmentation of the oral mucosa.

Some patients with leukaemia undergo haemopoietic stem cell transplantation and, as a result, approximately half will develop chronic graft versus host disease (cGVHD), about 100 days post transplant. This often affects the mouth, commonly manifesting as lichenoid lesions, frequently extensive and painful and difficult to manage effectively. Other oral manifestations include xerostomia, superficial mucoceles, pyogenic granulomas and oral mucosal changes consistent with those in systemic sclerosis. Immunosuppressants used in managing cGVHD may also produce oral adverse effects such as the gingival overgrowth associated with ciclosporin therapy, and they also render the patient susceptible to infection (oral herpetic and candidal involvement is common) and occasionally to malignancy. These patients are also likely to be receiving corticosteroids and this must be considered when planning dental treatment. Additionally, such patients may well be prescribed bisphosphonates as a bone-sparing prophylaxis and are at risk of osteochemonecrosis of the jaw, particularly following invasive dental procedures such as dental extraction.

Thrombocytopaenias

Thrombocytopaenia may be due to failure of the bone marrow to produce platelets (e.g. in aplastic anaemia or marrow infiltration) or result from their excessive destruction (e.g. idiopathic [autoimmune] thrombocytopaenic purpura; ITP).

Idiopathic thrombocytopaenic purpura is a common cause of platelet deficiency.

Clinical features

These include:

- Petechiae/purpura
- Ecchymoses
- Epistaxis
- Postoperative haemorrhage.

Clinical signs

Thrombocytopaenic purpura presents with bleeding into the tissues (Figures 5.8 and 5.9).

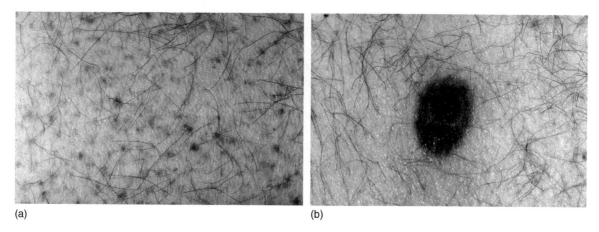

(a)   (b)

Figure 5.8 (a) and (b) Thrombocytopaenic purpura

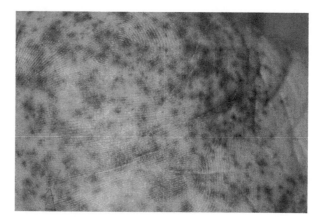

Figure 5.9 Thrombocytopaenic purpura

Diagnosis

● Full blood picture and platelet counts are indicated.

Management

● Corticosteroids or other immunosuppressives are the main treatments.
● Splenectomy is sometimes needed.

Oral health care relevance

● Submucous purpura and gingival bleeding may be seen.
● The main danger is haemorrhage on injections or surgery.

- Local haemostatic measures, desmopressin or tranexamic acid or topical administration of platelet concentrates can help.
- Platelets can be replaced or supplemented pre-operatively by platelet-rich plasma (PRP) transfusions given within 6–24 hours of their collection.
  - Regional local anaesthetic block injections can be given if the platelet levels are above 30×10^9/L.
  - Simple dentoalveolar surgery can usually be performed if platelet levels are above 50×10^9/L.
- Splenectomy predisposes to infections, typically with pneumococci rather than oral streptococci, so antimicrobial prophylaxis is not generally recommended.
- Drugs that damage platelets (such as NSAIDs) should be avoided.

6

Mental health conditions

Anxiety and stress

Anxiety is an unpleasant emotional state characterised by a subjective experience of fear and a variety of physical symptoms in response to a real or perceived threat. This is a normal response to stress and optimum levels can be beneficial, but stress can result in raised blood levels of 'stress hormones' – mainly the adrenal hormones cortisol, epinephrine (adrenaline) and norepinephrine (noradrenaline). These hormones influence a wide range of physiological functions and can result in disease. Cortisol is essential for the body at times of stress and serum levels exhibit a natural rise in the morning and fall at night. If this diurnal rhythm is disturbed, serum electrolyte balance, blood glucose control and stress responses are affected. While short-term elevations of cortisol are beneficial physiologically, chronically elevated levels result in Cushing syndrome.

Clinical features

Overwhelming autonomic activity can cause several physical effects. Sympathetic activity via the release of catecholamines causes apprehension, tachycardia, hyperventilation, hypertension, sweating, tremor, dilated pupils and dry mouth. Parasympathetic activity may lead to involuntary defaecation and urinary incontinence.

Clinical signs

The lines shown in Figure 6.1 on the nails (Beau lines), which are particularly distinct, are thought to result from the temporary cessation of growth of the nail plate following the death of a spouse and the related anxiety, stress and grief suffered. Nails with Beau lines are characterised by horizontal lines of light or darkened cells +/– linear depressions. This may also be caused by trauma, illness, malnutrition or any major metabolic condition, chemotherapy or other damaging event, and is the result of any interruption in the protein formation of the nail plate. Arsenic poisoning may also produce white lines and ridges in the nails.

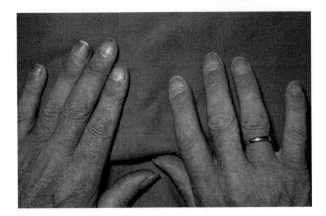

Figure 6.1   Beau lines resulting from stress

Diagnosis

Pathological anxiety may be difficult to diagnose and requires careful consideration of an individual's personal history and presenting clinical features. A
psychiatric assessment may be appropriate, but underlying organic causes such
as hyperthyroidism and mitral valve prolapse should be excluded first.

Anxiety can be classified into the following diagnostic categories:

- Panic disorder: discrete attacks with no external stimulus
- Phobias: discrete attacks with stimuli
- Generalised anxiety disorder: a generalised persistent state of anxiety
- As a manifestation of other psychiatric disease such as depression.

Management

Treatment of anxiety and stress may require:

- Appropriate management of any underlying organic disease
- Lifestyle changes to reduce stressors and avoid precipitating factors
- Behavioural techniques
- Pharmacotherapy (anxiolytics such as benzodiazepines and β-blockers)
- Psychotherapy: this may be used to aid adjustment of lifestyle (supportive)
  or to explore patient conflicts and secondary gain (psychodynamic).

Oral health care relevance

See *Oral health care relevance* under *Depression*, p. 92.

Depression

Depression is a disorder of emotion characterised by a persistent low mood
and negative thinking. The lifetime risk for depression is approximately 10%,
with rates being doubled in women.

Depression can be triggered by adverse life events such as a bereavement or divorce, and onset is typically in the third decade of life.

Clinical features

Features of depression include a persistent lowering of mood and feelings of hopelessness, worthlessness, helplessness and guilt. Individuals also have a reduced level of enjoyment (anhedonia) and reduced cognitive function with impaired concentration.

Biological function is altered. Patients may exhibit: lack of energy, fatigue, reduced concentration, insomnia, early-morning awakening, oversleeping, loss of appetite and weight loss or gain. Depression may also manifest as chronic pain of 'unknown cause'. It may impact significantly on an individual's quality of life and lead to thoughts of, or even attempts at suicide.

Clinical signs

Attempts at suicide, such as hanging, are all too common. Figure 6.2 shows rope burns from a hanging attempt.

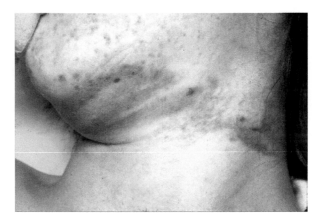

Figure 6.2   Rope burn from a suicide attempt

Diagnosis

Diagnosis of depression is dependent upon identifying:

- A persistent lowering of mood
- Alterations of biological function (as outlined above)
- Negative, pessimistic thoughts about themselves, the world and the future (Beck cognitive triad).

It is important to remember that depressed patients often present with other symptoms, and questionnaires to screen for thought and biological disturbances are therefore useful diagnostically.

Bipolar disorder is the term given to depression alternating with mania, which may amount to a psychosis. The various mood states in bipolar disorder may be regarded as a spectrum with severe depression at one end and mania at the other.

Management

The majority of patients with depression can be managed in the primary health-care setting by:

- Appropriate risk assessment for suicide and self-neglect: *psychiatric referral is needed if suicide risk is high* or the depression is severe and unresponsive to initial treatment
- Psychological techniques (cognitive-behaviour and supportive therapy)
- Pharmacotherapy (Table 6.1)
- Electroconvulsive therapy (ECT): for very severe cases where significant physical retardation or delusions (fixed, unshakeable, false beliefs) are present.

Table 6.1   Classification of anti-depressants

Class	Examples
Tricyclic anti-depressant (TCA)	Amitriptyline hydrochloride
Serotonin* norepinephrine reuptake inhibitor (SNRI)	Venlafaxine
Selective serotonin* reuptake inhibitor (SSRI)	Fluoxetine
Norepinephrine reuptake inhibitor (NRI)	Reboxetine
Norepinephrine and specific serotonergic agonist	Mirtazapine
Reversible inhibitor of monoamine oxidase A (RIMA)	Moclobemide
Monoamine oxidase inhibitor (MAOI)	Phenelzine

*Serotonin is 5-hydroxytryptamine (5-HT).

Oral health care relevance

- Anxious, stressed and depressed patients should be treated with an empathetic, unhurried and understanding approach.
- The use of intravenous, inhalational or other sedation techniques can be of great value in managing the very anxious or stressed patient.
- Orofacial manifestations of anxious or stressed patients include temporomandibular joint dysfunction, secondary to parafunctional jaw activity such as bruxism or tooth clenching; oral mucosal trauma such as cheek chewing; atypical (idiopathic) facial pain and oral dysaesthesias including burning mouth syndrome.
- Depressive illness may also be associated with cancerophobia and oral dysaesthesias although most patients with burning mouth syndrome show features of anxiety rather than depression.

- Somatoform disorder can be a feature of patients with anxiety or depression. Patients may describe various orofacial symptomatologies in great detail and the patient often believes that the commencement of the symptoms was related to some dental intervention. Symptoms are very diverse and commonly may include altered taste perception, dry mouth, halitosis, burning sensations, paraesthesiae, slimy sensations and fluid discharges.
- Cognitive behavioural therapy may be of benefit in managing the orofacial symptoms. Such patients may be best managed in conjunction with a liaison psychiatry service. Antidepressants may be indicated.
- Medication used to treat anxiety or depression may cause xerostomia. The tricyclic antidepressants are particularly notable in this regard.

Eating disorders

Dieting to a body weight lower than needed for health is common and heavily promoted in some activities (e.g. modelling), and by fashion trends and sales campaigns. Such eating disorders usually develop during adolescence or early adulthood, and most often in females, and they often coexist with other psychiatric problems such as depression, substance abuse and anxiety disorders.

Eating disorders can disturb growth and lead to endocrine problems, cardiac disease and renal failure, and can have such life-threatening health complications that they can be fatal.

Eating disorders include:

- Anorexia nervosa (self-imposed starvation)
- Bulimia nervosa (binge eating and dieting).

Clinical features

- Features of anorexia nervosa include:
  - Low body weight
  - Intense fear of gaining weight
  - Disturbance in body image
  - Attempting to control body weight
  - Peripheral cyanosis and coldness with bradycardia.
- Features of bulimia nervosa include:
  - Recurrent episodes of binge eating
  - Recurrent inappropriate compensatory behaviour in order to prevent weight gain, such as self-induced vomiting or misuse of laxatives, diuretics, enemas or other medications (purging).

Clinical signs

Bilateral painless parotid swelling may occur in sialosis (Figure 6.3) and, with xerostomia, in Sjögren syndrome and sarcoidosis.

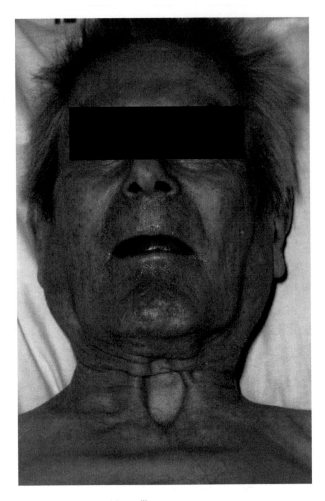

Figure 6.3   Bilateral painless parotid swelling

Whilst the cause of sialosis is often obscure, it may occur in malnutrition, including anorexia and bulimia, in alcoholism and in endocrine conditions such as pregnancy, diabetes mellitus, thyroid disease and acromegaly. It is thought to be associated with abnormal autonomic function of the salivary glands. Certain drugs such as isoprenaline, iodine derivatives and, rarely, chlorhexidine may also produce salivary gland swelling.

Diagnosis

- Diagnosis is on clinical grounds.

Management

Treatment may include:

- Medical care and monitoring
- Psychosocial interventions (cognitive-behavioural or interpersonal psychotherapy)
- Nutritional counselling
- Medication: selective serotonin reuptake inhibitors (SSRIs).

Oral health care relevance

- Tooth erosion may result from repeated vomiting.
- Parotid enlargement (sialosis) and angular stomatitis may develop.
- Palatal ulcers or abrasions may be caused by induced vomiting.

Schizophrenia

Schizophrenia is a chronic condition of complex aetiology characterised by dopamine overactivity in the mesolimbic pathways of the brain. It has a lifetime prevalence of approximately 1%.

Mood, thoughts and behaviour are disorganised and appear irrational and exaggerated. Disorders of perception (hallucinations) and thought (delusions) are common.

Clinical features

Acute schizophrenia typically presents in young individuals with positive symptoms (hallucinations, delusions and thought disorder). The person generally lacks insight and concern is initially raised by a friend or relative.

Chronic schizophrenia may present insidiously with negative symptoms (apathy, loss of affect and social withdrawal) and can thus be easily misdiagnosed. Disintegration of the individual's personality results in social isolation and withdrawal. Some patients are strikingly paranoid whilst others exhibit motor impairment (catatonia) or a mixture of emotional, behavioural and thought disturbances (hebephrenia).

Clinical signs

There are no specific signs of schizophrenia apart from behavioural but treatment can have adverse effects. Chlorpromazine can cause tardive dyskinesia, a not uncommon side effect, dry mouth and hyperpigmentation (Figure 6.4). It is typically grey/purple in colour and occurs especially on exposed skin surfaces. It arises as a consequence of photosensitivity as well as due to the deposition of coloured metabolites within the tissues.

Mucosal pigmentation due to chlorpromazine may also occur as shown here in association with a traumatic ulcer (Figure 6.5).

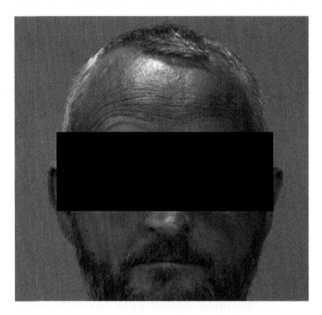

Figure 6.4 Hyperpigmentation as a result of taking chlorpromazine

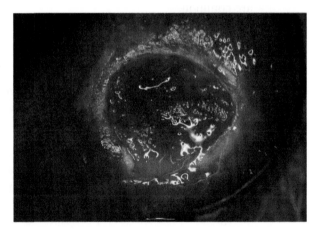

Figure 6.5 Traumatic ulcer with hyperpigmentation due to chlorpromazine

A variety of other drugs *unrelated* to mental health can also cause diffuse mucosal and skin pigmentation. These include the oral contraceptive, antimalarials, certain cytotoxics (cyclophosphamide), amiodarone, gold, minocycline and phenothiazines. Generalised intrinsic pigmentation of the oral mucosa includes variations of normal as in racial pigmentation, pigmentary incontinence induced by inflammatory conditions as in lichen planus and tobacco smoking. Addison disease is a further cause.

Diagnosis

The diagnosis of schizophrenia is complex and should be made by an experienced psychiatrist. The diagnostic criteria for schizophrenia vary but include the recognition of Schneider's first rank symptoms:

- Auditory hallucinations: thought echo or voices talking about the patient in the third person
- Passivity: the feeling of being controlled by external forces
- Thought insertion or withdrawal
- Thought broadcasting
- Delusions
- Hallucinations.

Management

Treatment of schizophrenia includes:

- Assessment of patient risk to themselves or others; individuals may require acute psychiatric admission under the Mental Health Act
- Supportive therapy via community psychiatric services
- Long-term psychotherapy
- Anti-psychotic drug therapy, nowadays more with atypical anti-psychotics than chlorpromazine (Table 6.2).

Table 6.2 Anti-psychotic drugs used to treat schizophrenia

Drug class	Examples
Atypical anti-psychotics	Clozapine
Piperazine phenothiazines	Prochlorperazine
Phenothiazines	Chlorpromazine
Butyrophenones	Haloperidol
Thioxanthines	Flupenthixol
Diphenylbutylpiperidines	Pimozide

Oral health care relevance

- Dental management of the patient may be complicated by inappropriate behaviour or bizarre oral symptomatology.
- Anti-psychotic drugs can produce dyskinesias and xerostomia which can be severe. Additionally, chlorpromazine may produce grey/violaceous mucocutaneous pigmentation.

7

Neurological conditions

Bell palsy

Bell palsy as described by Dr Charles Bell in the 19th century is a lower motor neurone facial paralysis (seventh cranial nerve) where no local or systemic cause can be identified. Bell palsy, however, is now recognised to be mainly due to infection with herpes simplex virus (HSV).

Similar features may be seen after other infections – herpesvirus infections (e.g. VZV, CMV, EBV), influenza, retroviruses (e.g. HIV and HTLV-1) and others such as Lyme disease (*Borrelia burgdorferi*) – as well as in diabetes, connective tissue diseases, granulomatous disorders and multiple sclerosis.

Clinical features

- Acute unilateral facial paralysis, maximal within 48 hours.
- Occasionally hyperacusis (oversensitivity to sound, due to loss of function of nerve to stapedius), or loss of taste (chorda tympani) on the anterior tongue, or changes in salivation/lacrimation.
- No other neurological deficits.

Clinical signs

Bell palsy impairs the ability to smile (Figure 7.1). On asking the patient to close the eyes, the eye on the affected side also rolls upwards and outwards – Bell sign. The entire side of the face is paralysed, whilst in upper motor neurone involvement (such as a stroke), there is sparing of the forehead because of bilateral innervation and the patient is able to wrinkle the forehead. Differential diagnosis of Bell palsy should include: stroke, brainstem lesions, multiple sclerosis, mononeuritis, compression by tumours such as acoustic neuroma or parotid tumour, facial trauma, Ramsay Hunt syndrome, and Melkersson–Rosenthal syndrome.

Melkersson–Rosenthal syndrome is a rare condition consisting of a triad of intermittent facial nerve paralysis, persistent or recurring lip or facial swelling, and a fissured tongue (Figure 7.2). The aetiology of this condition is unknown but it may be related to Crohn disease or the related orofacial granulomatosis. The orofacial swelling usually manifests as pronounced lip enlargement. It may

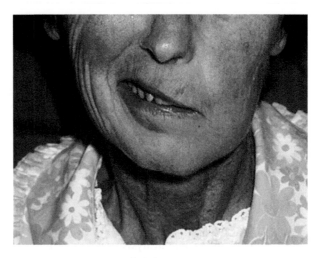

Figure 7.1　Inability to smile in Bell palsy

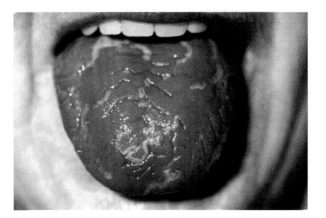

Figure 7.2　Fissured tongue in Melkersson–Rosenthal syndrome

or may not affect both lips, may be tender or erythematous and shows granulomas on biopsy. The presence of a fissured tongue in association with these other features is diagnostic of the condition. The facial paralysis is clinically indistinguishable from Bell palsy, and it may be an inconsistent and intermittent finding with spontaneous resolution.

Diagnosis

- Bell palsy must be distinguished from upper motor neurone (UMN) palsy such as in a stroke.
- Electromyography (EMG) can confirm facial nerve damage and determine its severity but is rarely needed.
- If paralysis is progressive, imaging of the internal acoustic canal, cerebellopontine angle and mastoid may be needed to exclude a tumour.

Management

- Eighty five percent of patients totally recover spontaneously within a few weeks. Incomplete paralysis is a favourable prognostic sign.
- Hyperacusis, severe taste impairment and/or diminished lacrimation or salivation, especially in older, diabetic or hypertensive patients are bad prognostic signs.
- The cornea should meantime be protected with an eye pad.
- Active treatment includes:
  - Anti-inflammatory medication (prednisolone)
  - Anti-viral medication (aciclovir or famciclovir)
  - Facial massage to help try and prevent permanent contractures.

Oral health care relevance

- Facial palsy may lead to poor oral cleansing and accumulation of food debris and plaque on the affected side.
- Saliva may leak from the affected side and cause angular stomatitis.

Cerebrovascular accident

A stroke or cerebrovascular accident (CVA) is a common cause of death and disability worldwide, especially in older people. A stroke is the syndrome of rapidly developing signs of focal or global disturbance of cerebral functions, lasting greater than 24 hours or leading to death. It may be preceded by a transient ischaemic attack (TIA), which by definition is characterised by focal cerebral and neurological features that resolve completely within 24 hours. A reversible ischaemic neurological deficit (RIND) is similar to a TIA but persists for more than 24 hours. Unlike a stroke, recovery from a RIND is complete with no detectable residual neurological deficit.

Strokes result from cerebral ischaemia and infarction in 80% of cases, the most common cause being cerebral atheroma in which plaque rupture results in arterial occlusion or thrombosis. Intracerebral or subarachnoid haemorrhages, by causing pressure and ischaemic damage of adjacent structures, account for nearly 20% of strokes. Finally, an embolism from the left side of the heart (a potential complication of chronic atrial fibrillation) may rarely obstruct cerebral blood flow.

Risk factors for CVA include:

- Preceding TIA or previous stroke
- Old age
- Hypertension
- Heart disease (atrial fibrillation, ischaemic or valvular heart disease)
- Diabetes mellitus
- Hypercholesterolaemia
- Smoking

- Alcohol
- Obesity
- Hyperviscosity syndromes, prothrombotic and haemorrhagic states.

Clinical features

The clinical manifestations of CVA vary according to the duration, severity and pattern of cerebral ischaemia. Typical features include: visual deterioration, speech disturbance, hemiplegia (loss of voluntary movement of the opposite side of the body to the cerebral lesion), and impaired level of consciousness progressing to coma or death. Approximately 45% of people with a stroke die within a month. Of survivors, 40% have mild disability, 40% require special care, 10% recover completely and 10% require long-term hospitalisation.

Clinical signs

Pressure sores (bed sores) may complicate stroke if care is not adequate (Figure 7.3).

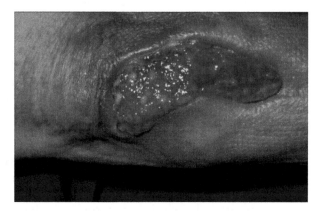

Figure 7.3   Pressure sore

Diagnosis

The diagnosis of CVA is essentially a clinical one and is based upon a history and clinical features suggestive of neurological deficit. It is important to assess risk factors for cerebrovascular disease including co-morbid medical conditions. The following investigations may be indicated:

- Computed tomography (CT) or magnetic resonance imaging (MRI): to localise the site of and assess the degree of cerebral damage
- Cardiac investigations: to screen for arrhythmias and valvular heart disease

- Carotid duplex scans: to assess arterial blood flow to the brain
- Cerebral arteriography: to identify a source of haemorrhage
- Clotting, thrombophilia and vasculitic screens.

Management

Virtually all stroke victims should be admitted to hospital for assessment and management, as early treatment in a dedicated stroke unit lowers patient mortality and morbidity. Supportive care includes:

- Protection of the airway including appropriate ventilatory support
- If swallowing is impaired, the patient should be kept nil by mouth and a nasogastric tube may be placed to reduce the risk of aspiration pneumonia
- Pressure sensitive nursing to avoid the development of pressure sores
- Urinary catheterisation and incontinence pads if urethral and anal sphincteric reflexes are impaired
- Physiotherapy to reduce muscle wasting and disuse atrophy
- Speech and language assessment
- Occupational therapy for long-term rehabilitation.

Medical treatment may include:

- Nimodipine (a calcium antagonist): to reduce intracranial vasospasm
- Aspirin and anticoagulants for non-haemorrhagic strokes
- Thrombolytic therapy: streptokinase or recombinant tissue plasminogen activator (rTPA) if administered early may re-establish cerebral blood flow to the affected area and thus prevent or limit the extent of cerebral infarction
- Emergency neurosurgery to clip a leaking aneurysm in the case of a subarachnoid haemorrhage or evacuate a large intracerebral bleed. Carotid endarterectomy to remove atheroma from the carotid arteries in an attempt to improve blood flow to the cerebral arteries may eventually be indicated but only after full recovery from the initial event.

Oral health care relevance

- The dental management of stroke patients depends on the nature and degree of functional impairment sustained. This may include physical disability as well as cognitive impairment with difficulty in communication.
- Dental treatment should be provided in as stress-free a fashion as possible with short appointments, ideally avoiding early mornings as blood pressure tends to be higher at this time.
- Gag and swallowing reflexes may be impaired and therefore effective aspiration is important (particularly if the patient is to be sedated).
- There may be a bleeding tendency if the patient has been anti-coagulated, and this must be considered if invasive dental treatment is planned.

- Considerations applicable to patients with hypertension are equally relevant to those who have had a cerebrovascular accident.
- Orofacial manifestations include facial palsy, which may contribute to poor oral hygiene, further compromised if manual dexterity is impaired by the stroke.
- Stroke may occur in the dental surgery and members of the dental team should be aware of its clinical presentation (viz. sudden loss of consciousness with hemiplegia), and emergency management. The dental team must ensure airway patency and call for an ambulance.

Epilepsy

A seizure (fit) is a convulsion or transient disturbance in consciousness, which is caused by abnormal increased cerebral electrical activity. Epilepsy is a predisposition for recurrent seizures. Epilepsy affects approximately 1% of the adult population and may reflect underlying cerebral pathology (injury, tumours or infections). Cerebral hypoxia, metabolic disturbances (hypoglycaemia or hyperglycaemia) and drugs (neuroleptic drugs, barbiturates, alcohol, opioids, cocaine and amphetamines) may predispose to epilepsy.

Clinical features

The clinical presentation of epilepsy is variable and classification is complex (Table 7.1).

The majority of epileptic seizures are idiopathic but, in some instances, may be precipitated by: food or sleep deprivation, concurrent illness, metabolic disturbances, sensory stimuli (flashing lights) or drugs (prescribed or illicit).

Table 7.1   Classification and clinical features of epilepsy

Type	Sub-type	Clinical features
Generalised seizures	Tonic–clonic (grand mal)	Loss of consciousness Tonic phase Clonic phase Tongue biting Incontinence Seizure lasts <5 minutes
	Absence seizure (petit mal)	Brief period of unresponsiveness Duration of absences <30 seconds
Partial seizures	Simple (Jacksonian epilepsy)	No impairment of consciousness Motor, sensory and autonomic features
	Complex (temporal lobe epilepsy)	Impaired consciousness Automatic repetitive acts

Clinical signs

Trauma to oral tissues is common, as in Figure 7.4, where the lip was bitten. Trauma to the maxillary incisors in particular is common, as in Figure 7.5, where the incisor has been subsequently inadequately restored.

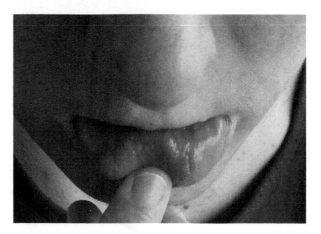

Figure 7.4   Bitten lip as a consequence of a seizure

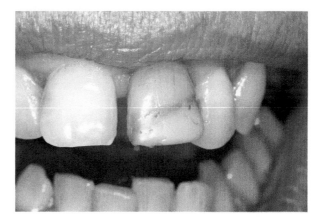

Figure 7.5   Incisor damaged and non-vital after an epileptic seizure

Phenytoin anti-convulsant therapy may produce gingival swelling, or swelling of the oral mucosa (Figure 7.6).

Most epilepsy is idiopathic and there are no obvious external signs, but occasionally there are overt signs such as café au lait spots due to neurofibromatosis (NF), a common neurological genetic condition underlying fits (Figure 7.7). The development of NF is linked to increased concentrations of nerve growth stimulating activity. The disease tends to change and develop with time

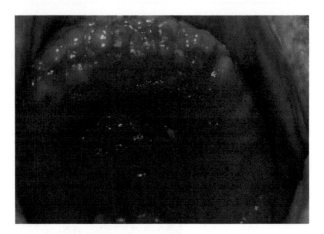

Figure 7.6   Swelling resulting from phenytoin therapy

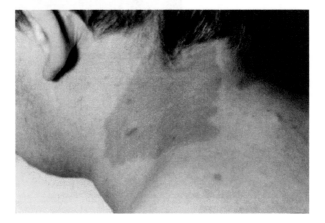

Figure 7.7   Café au lait spots

and some patients may only have cutaneous manifestations, while others have life-threatening or severely disfiguring complications with or without learning disability. When neurofibromas increase in size or cause pain, malignant transformation should be suspected, and excision or biopsy should be performed. Acoustic neuromas and tumours that cause tinnitus and vertigo should be excised with great caution. Any signs of epilepsy should be investigated, and responsible tumours should be removed.

Diagnosis

The diagnosis of epilepsy involves:

- A history of recurrent seizures without an obvious underlying cause
- Detailed neuromuscular assessment

- Blood investigations to screen for infection and metabolic abnormalities (full blood count, liver and renal profiles, inflammatory markers)
- An electroencephalogram (EEG) to measure brain electrical activity
- Computed tomography (CT) and magnetic resonance imaging (MRI) to screen for cerebral pathology
- Lumbar puncture and cerebrospinal fluid (CSF) analysis to exclude cerebral and meningeal infection.

Management

Management of epilepsy includes:

- Patient education, in particular regarding how to avoid damage to the patient and others
- Identification and avoidance of precipitating or trigger factors
- Treatment of any identifiable predisposing pathology or disease
- Prophylactic anticonvulsant therapy (Table 7.2).

Table 7.2 Anticonvulsant treatment of epilepsy

Type of epilepsy	Medication	Adverse effects*
Tonic–clonic seizure	Phenytoin	Rashes
	Carbamazepine	Blood dyscrasias
	Sodium valproate	Liver impairment
Absence seizure	Sodium valproate	Liver impairment
	Ethosuximide	Sleep disturbance
Partial seizures	Carbamazepine	Blood dyscrasias
	Sodium valproate	Liver impairment

*All can cause drowsiness and ataxia.

Oral health care relevance

- Oral mucosal trauma and damage to the teeth or jaws may occur during epileptic seizures.
- Drug-induced gingival overgrowth, secondary to the use of phenytoin.
- Anticonvulsants may also produce erythema multiforme in susceptible patients. These drugs may also reduce absorption of dietary folic acid, resulting in folate deficiency that predisposes patients to candidosis and aphthous-like ulcers.
- Drug interactions may occur between anticonvulsants and antimicrobials including metronidazole, azoles and doxycycline.
- Midazolam should only be used in well-controlled epileptic patients in the primary care setting, i.e. patients having less than one attack per month.

- The use of flumazenil should be avoided in the epileptic patient.
- The clinician should ensure that a detailed history of the nature, degree of control and frequency of the seizures is obtained, whether the patient has an aura prior to an attack and ascertain whether the medication has been taken on the day of the planned dental treatment.
- The dental team must be conversant with the management of epileptic attacks in the dental surgery.

Multiple sclerosis

Multiple sclerosis (MS) is the most common neurological disease of young adults. The aetiology of MS remains unknown. Twice as common in men as in women, it is thought to be an autoimmune disease directed against myelin sheath proteins in genetically susceptible individuals. It is a chronic relapsing disorder characterised by the formation of 'plaques' (areas of demyelination) throughout the central nervous system (CNS).

Clinical features

The clinical features of MS depend on the area of CNS affected and may include:

- Numbness, weakness or paralysis in a limb
- Visual disturbances and pain on eye movement (optic neuritis)
- Brief pain, tingling or electric-shock sensations
- Tremor, lack of coordination or unsteady gait
- Urinary incontinence, constipation and sexual dysfunction
- Cognitive changes (memory loss and impaired concentration).

Clinical signs

Optic atrophy is a serious complication (Figure 7.8).

Diagnosis

The diagnostic hallmark of MS is a series of neurological deficits distributed in time and space not explained by any other causes. Diagnosis is assisted by:

- Magnetic resonance imaging (MRI): to identify demyelinating disease
- Delayed visual evoked response potentials (VEPs)
- Cerebrospinal fluid examination: may demonstrate a raised white blood cell count, increased protein concentration and oligoclonal bands.

Management

Multiple sclerosis is a chronic disabling disease and management therefore

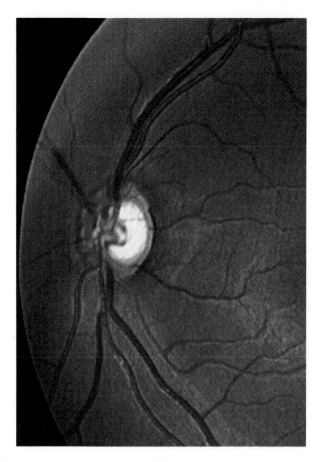

Figure 7.8 Optic atrophy in multiple sclerosis

requires a multidisciplinary team with close liaison between patient, doctors, therapists and carers. Care may include:

- Physical and occupational therapy
- Counselling: the Multiple Sclerosis Society provides information and support for patients and relatives
- Corticosteroids: promote remission in acute episodes but do not influence long-term prognosis
- Subcutaneous interferon beta may reduce the relapse rate of MS but is expensive and adverse effects (flu-like symptoms) are common
- Muscle relaxants (baclofen, dantrolene and benzodiazepines): reduce pain caused by spastic muscle paralysis
- Alemtuzumab: may halt progression of early MS and may effect repair of damaged nerves, thereby reversing disability.

Oral health care relevance

- Patients present with varying levels of disability, and their dental needs will therefore be dependent on severity and nature of the disease process.

- Patient mobility may compromise access to the dental surgery.
- Physical disability can also result in poor oral hygiene and carers will be required to help the patient in this regard.
- Patients with severe MS should not be treated supine as this can compromise their respiration.
- Patients may be taking corticosteroids and this must be taken into account when planning invasive procedures.
- There is a theoretical risk of nitrous oxide producing further demyelination and therefore its use is best avoided.

Multiple sclerosis should be considered as a possible diagnosis in young patients with symptoms suggestive of trigeminal neuralgia and those with unexplainable recurrent or persistent orofacial paraesthesias or facial palsies.

Dementia

Dementia is an acquired and progressive loss of intellect, memory and social abilities without clouding of consciousness. The prevalence increases with age, being rare before 60 years of age, and affecting approximately 20% of those over 80 years. Causes of dementia are shown in Table 7.3.

Table 7.3   Types of dementia

Common	Uncommmon causes
Alzheimer disease	Brain-occupying lesion
Multi-infarct dementia	Chronic traumatic encephalopathy
Lewy body dementia	Creutzfeldt–Jakob disease
	HIV infection/AIDS
	Hypothyroidism
	Huntington chorea
	Syphilis
	Vitamin B12 deficiency
	Wernicke–Korsakoff syndrome

Alzheimer disease is the most common form of dementia and is a neurodegenerative disease that results in progressive cognitive impairment. The pathological hallmarks of Alzheimer disease are brain neurofibrillary tangles and argentophile plaques consisting of dying neurons clustered close to deposits of amyloid. HSV has been implicated.

Clinical features

Early symptoms of dementia are loss of short-term (recent) memory and an inability to perform previously simple tasks. In advanced dementia individuals may be disoriented in time, place and person. Progressive impairment of memory, cognitive function and personality leads to social difficulties and self-neglect. Features of anxiety and depression may also be present.

Clinical signs

There are no other specific signs apart from sometimes those associated with neglect, but chronic exposure to the heat from a domestic fire may cause erythema ab igne (Figure 7.9).

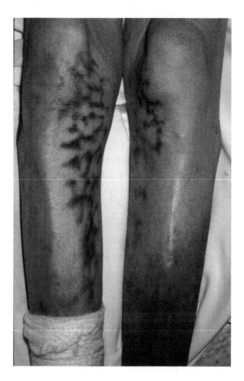

Figure 7.9 Erythema ab igne

Diagnosis

The diagnosis of dementia depends on evidence of a progressive decline in cognitive function in the absence of focal neurological deficits and the exclusion of other organic disease. Investigations include:

- Clinical assessment of mental state and social function
- Full blood count, renal and liver profiles
- Vitamin B12 and folate levels
- Syphilis serology
- Septic screen
- Brain computed tomography (CT) or magnetic resonance imaging (MRI).

Management

Patients with dementia should be managed in the community if possible although a detailed assessment by a psychogeriatrician is often needed. Treatment may involve:

- Management of concurrent medical problems which may make dementia worse (e.g. chest or urinary tract infections or malnutrition)
- Acetylcholinesterase inhibitors (donepezil [Aricept], rivastigmine, or galantamine): to slow intellectual deterioration
- Sedatives and antidepressants: to help manage associated anxiety and depression
- Social services, with supportive interventions for both patients and carers. Long-term residential or nursing home care may become a necessity.

Oral health care relevance

- In order to address behavioural issues, a sympathetic approach will be required at all times.
- Consideration must be given to the timing of appointments together with an understanding that patients may forget to attend.
- Treatment must be tailored to meet the patient's oral and general health needs.
- Access to high quality dental care with particular regard to the assessment of specific dental need can also be an issue especially if the patient has some degree of physical disability as may well be the case.
- Additionally sedation or general anaesthetic services may be required.
- Compliance with advice will be an issue and, if at all possible, the patient's carer should be informed of all procedures that are to be undertaken, keeping in mind issues of consent and autonomy. In more advanced cases, the carer should be advised on how best to help the patient with regard to personal oral care and to supervise the patient's medication where appropriate.
- If there are significant behavioural issues, the patient may be taking psychoactive drugs that are likely to produce xerostomia, contributing further to the patient's dental needs.
- In the past, older patients were frequently edentulous, however with improvements in oral health this is no longer the case and therefore treating people with dementia can pose a significant restorative challenge.

8

Osteoarticular conditions

Osteoarthritis

Osteoarthritis (OA) is the most common type of arthritis and most important cause of locomotor disability. It is characterised by degeneration of articular cartilage with compensatory thickening of the exposed underlying bone and development of peri-articular cysts, which collapse and, together with continued peripheral bone proliferation, cause progressive joint deformity. Risk factors for OA include:

- Age (usually over 45 years)
- Gender – females more commonly affected
- Genetic predisposition
- Obesity
- Malformed joints (hereditary or acquired)
- Occupation (athletes).

Osteoarthritis may affect any joint, but especially affects frequently used, weight-bearing or traumatised joints – such as those in the fingers, hips, knees, lower back and feet.

Clinical features

Features include: joint pain with stiffness, joint deformity, crepitus, effusion, loss of joint flexibility and reduced function. Bony exostoses may develop on the fingers and at the thumb base.

Clinical signs

In the hands, bony swellings and deformity affect the distal interphalangeal joints (Figures 8.1 and 8.2; best seen on the middle finger in Figure 8.1) where they are termed Heberden nodes. Similar swelling of the proximal interphalangeal joints are called Bouchard nodes (see Figure 8.1: ring finger).

Diagnosis

The diagnosis of OA is usually on clinical grounds, the absence of systemic features (in contrast to rheumatoid arthritis), supported by imaging showing the characteristic radiographic features of:

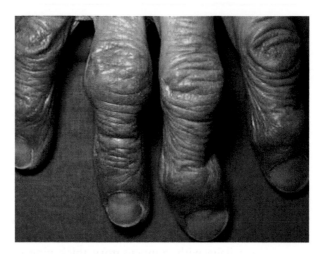

Figure 8.1   Heberden and Bouchard nodes

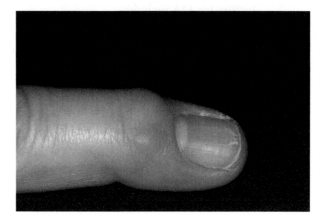

Figure 8.2   Heberden nodes

- Narrowing of the joint space
- Marginal osteophyte formation (lipping)
- Subchondral bone sclerosis
- Peri-articular bone 'cysts' (rounded areas of radiolucency just beneath the joint surface)
- Joint deformity.

Management

Management aims in OA include:

- Patient education
- Pain reduction
- Optimisation of mobility and function
- Prevention of further joint deterioration.

General management of patients with OA may include:

- Information and advice, including how to access community support
- Weight reduction
- Appropriate footwear and chiropody
- Exercise and walking aids to encourage mobility and improve muscle strength
- Heat and cold application.

Medical treatment of OA may include:

- Topical analgesics and counter-irritants (e.g. capsaicin cream)
- Non-steroidal anti-inflammatory drugs
- Glucosamine
- Aspiration of joint effusions
- Intra-articular injections with a corticosteroid or joint lubricant (sodium hyaluronate).

Surgical treatment of OA may include:

- Arthroscopy: permits removal of joint fragments that may be contributing to pain, crepitus or mechanical symptoms such as 'locking'
- Joint replacement: although the hip joint is most commonly replaced, prosthetic replacements are available for shoulder, elbow, finger, knee and ankle joints
- Surgery to correct bony deformities: bones may be fused permanently to improve joint stability and reduce pain.

Oral health care relevance

- The temporomandibular joint may be affected in some patients, but it is not usually symptomatic.
- There is no indication to give antibiotic prophylaxis to patients who have received prosthetic joints as a consequence of osteoarthritic joint damage.
- Compromised mobility may complicate patient access to dental care.
- A disease complex comprising histological evidence of sialadenitis in minor salivary glands, osteoarthritis and xerostomia (SOX) has been described. However, these features are all frequently occurring and may represent a coincidental relationship rather than being truly interrelated aetiologically.

Rheumatoid arthritis

Rheumatoid arthritis (RA) affects women approximately three times as frequently as men, typically between the ages of 30 and 40 years. It is a multi-system immunologically mediated disease, occurring in genetically predisposed individuals (*HLA-DR4* genotype).

The aetiology is unclear but it is autoimmune and characterised by the presence of rheumatoid factor (RF) – an IgM antibody directed against abnormal

IgG – which forms immune complexes and leads to activation of complement, synovial inflammation and destructive joint disease.

Clinical features

Rheumatoid arthritis is a chronic symmetrical polyarthritis mainly of the small joints of the wrists, hands and feet and is characterised by increasing joint stiffness – worst in the morning – and aching, swelling, redness, tenderness and limitation of movement of affected joints.

Eventually, hand joints become spindle-shaped as a result of joint swelling with muscle wasting on either side. Ulnar deviation of the fingers may develop. Since the wrists, elbows, knees and ankles are often involved, patients become increasingly disabled. The cervical spine is involved in 30% of individuals and may be complicated by atlanto-axial subluxation. Non-articular features of RA are variable and include:

- Weight loss
- Fever
- Malaise
- Lymph node enlargement
- Subcutaneous rheumatoid nodules
- Palmar erythema and cutaneous vasculitis
- Sjögren syndrome
- Scleritis and episcleritis
- Pleural effusions and rheumatoid lung disease
- Pericarditis, mitral valve disease and cardiac conduction abnormalities
- Mononeuritis, carpal tunnel syndrome and peripheral neuropathy
- Normochromic normocytic anaemia of chronic disease
- Felty syndrome (seropositive RA, splenomegaly and neutropaenia).

Clinical signs

Rheumatoid arthritis typically involves the metacarpophalangeal and proximal interphalangeal joints symmetrically (Figure 8.3). Advanced disease produces various hand changes, including ulnar deviation and muscle wasting (both shown), swan neck deformity 'Z-shaped' thumb and Boutonniere deformity. A rheumatoid nodule is shown just below the elbow. Their presence confirms a diagnosis of seropositive rheumatoid disease.

Wasting of the thenar eminence (the muscle bulk at the base of the thumb) (Figure 8.4) is typical of carpal tunnel syndrome, caused by pressure on the median nerve as it passes through the enclosed space of the wrist (the carpal tunnel). Patients complain of tingling, which is typically worse at night and can disturb sleep; they are often awake and try to relieve symptoms by shaking the hand. This is caused mainly by RA, but other identifiable causes include pregnancy (the latter being both common and reversible after delivery), diabetes, hypothyroidism and acromegaly.

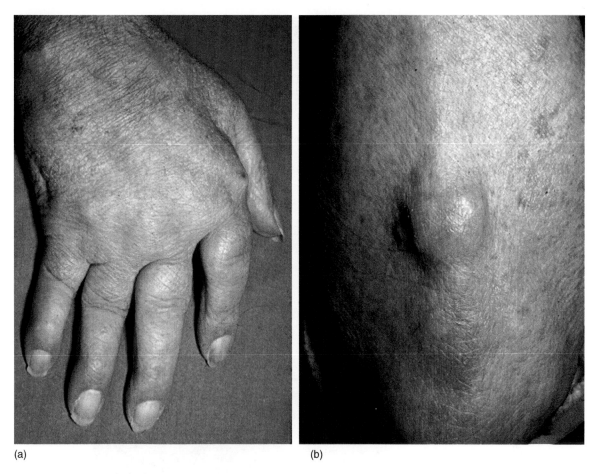

(a)   (b)

Figure 8.3   (a) Metacarpophalangeal and proximal interphalangeal joints affected by rheumatoid arthritis; (b) rheumatoid nodule

Diagnosis

The diagnosis of RA is based on clinical features and:

- Raised inflammatory markers (erythrocyte sedimentation rate [ESR] and C-reactive protein [CRP])
- Positive rheumatoid factor (RF present in 95% of cases).

Radiographic features of RA include:

- Widening of the joint space (early stages)
- Narrowing of the joint spaces (later stages)
- Joint erosion (an early sign), destruction and deformity
- Peri-articular osteoporosis.

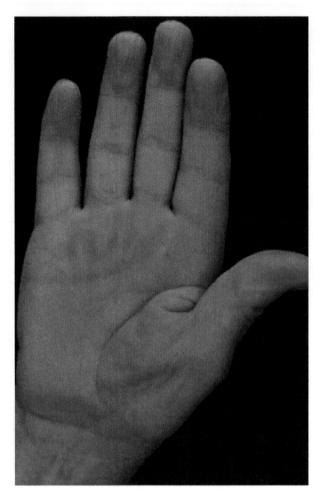

Figure 8.4   Wasting of the thenar eminence

Management

Management of RA includes:

- General supportive measures such as splints and appliances to facilitate mobility, reduce pain and preserve function
- Drugs:
    - Non-steroidal anti-inflammatory drugs and simple analgesics
    - Corticosteroids: may be given via intra-articular injections in acute phases
    - Disease modifying anti-rheumatic drugs (DMARDs): sulfasalazine, gold, penicillamine, minocycline and anti-malarials slow disease progression. Methotrexate, azathioprine, ciclosporin and cyclophosphamide are used for severe disease
    - Biological response modifiers: anti-tumour necrosis factor (anti-TNF) agents (infliximab and etanercept)
- Surgery: indicated for replacement of severely damaged joints.

Oral health care relevance

- Secondary Sjögren syndrome may complicate approximately 50% of cases and is the main orofacial manifestation.
- Radiological changes in the temporomandibular joint (TMJ) are frequent, including condylar erosions, but symptoms are uncommon.
- Subluxation of the atlanto-axial joint or fracture of the odontoid peg is a potentially catastrophic complication of sudden neck extension. As it may cause death or paralysis, care is required in positioning the patient, avoiding abrupt movements of the neck.
- Anaemia may complicate rheumatoid arthritis, and its treatment with non-steroidal anti-inflammatory drugs may also predispose to prolonged bleeding.
- Disease modifying anti-rheumatoid drugs (e.g. methotrexate) produce a degree of immunosuppression and a minority of patients will be on corticosteroid therapy. The risks of infection and possible need for steroid boosting should be considered when providing dental treatment.

Gout

In gout, joint uric acid crystal deposits result in release of lysosomal enzymes from polymorphonuclear leukocytes, causing acute inflammation.

- Primary gout is an inborn error of metabolism causing raised serum uric acid levels (hyperuricaemia).
- Secondary gout is usually caused by cell breakdown from drug treatment or radiotherapy of myeloproliferative diseases.

Clinical features

- Acute gout causes sudden and intensely severe joint pain, usually in the big toe (Figure 8.5), associated with fever, leukocytosis and raised serum uric acid levels. It can usually readily be differentiated from other forms of arthritis (Table 8.1).

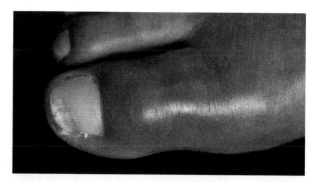

Figure 8.5   Acute gout

Table 8.1   Comparison of main forms of arthritis

	Osteoarthritis	Rheumatoid arthritis	Gout
Age of onset	Late middle age or older	Typically middle age, but juvenile variant may also occur	Late middle age or older
Pain and disability	+	++	++
Main joints affected	Weight-bearing or frequently used joints (hip, spine, knee, fingers)	Bilateral and usually symmetrical distribution; typically the proximal interphalangeal and metacarpophalangeal joints of the hands and corresponding joints of the feet	Big toe usually (may be ankle, heel, instep, knee, wrist, elbow, fingers or spine)
Clinical inflammation over joints	–	+	+
Joint deformities	Heberden or Bouchard nodes	Swelling and deviations e.g. ulnar deviation, 'Z-shaped' deviation of thumb, 'swan neck' and Boutonniere deformities of the fingers	Swelling and possibly tophi
Morning stiffness	Some	Pronounced	Some
Systemic problems, malaise, fatigue	–	+	+
Erythrocyte sedimentation rate	Normal	Raised	Often raised
Rheumatoid factor	–	+ usually	–

- Chronic (tophaceous) gout may cause tophi (masses of urate crystals which, in joints, interfere with function and also destroy bone and cartilage).
- Renal disease (gouty nephropathy), unless treated, can lead to fatal renal failure.

Clinical signs

Gouty tophi (Figure 8.6) are caused by deposition of sodium urate crystals in soft tissues.

Diagnosis

- Blood chemistry shows raised uric acid levels.
- Secondary gout should be investigated for the underlying disorder.

Management

- Colchicine and indometacin relieve an acute attack.
- Allopurinol reduces the frequency of acute gouty attacks (but should not be commenced until some weeks after an acute episode).
- Probenecid or sulfinpyrazone can help by increasing uric acid excretion.

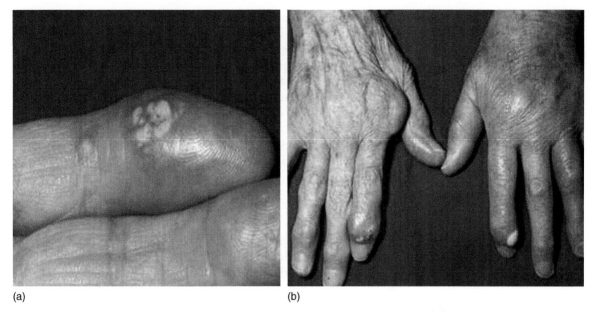

(a)   (b)

Figure 8.6 (a) and (b) Gouty tophi

Oral health care relevance

- Gout affects the temporomandibular joint only rarely.
- Allopurinol, which is used to treat gout, may produce lichenoid reactions.
- The incidence of rashes with ampicillin, but not other penicillin allergies, is greater in patients on allopurinol.
- Aspirin is contraindicated as it interferes with uricosuric drugs.

Sjögren syndrome

Sjögren syndrome (SS) is an autoimmune exocrinopathy, lymphocytes infiltrating lachrymal, salivary and other exocrine glands and causing acinar destruction. Females constitute 90% of cases.

- Primary SS is the association of dry mouth (xerostomia) with dry eyes (keratoconjunctivitis sicca) in the absence of any other connective tissue disease.
- Secondary SS is the association of dry mouth (xerostomia) with dry eyes (keratoconjunctivitis sicca) and a connective tissue disease, usually rheumatoid arthritis.

Clinical features

- Sjögren syndrome is a multisystem disease.
- Marked lethargy is an almost universal symptom, the cause of which is poorly understood.

- Raynaud phenomenon (arterial vasospasm in the hands and feet) is common.
- Ocular involvement may include dryness (which can cause keratocon-junctivitis sicca that can impair sight) and swelling of the lachrymal glands.
- Oral involvement may include dryness, which may be so severe as to cause functional disturbances, leading to difficulties in eating, taste perception, swallowing and speech, and swelling of the major salivary glands. This may be due to a variety of causes – obstructive, inflammatory, infective or neoplastic.
- Other mucosal surfaces, including the vagina and nasal mucosae, may be dry.
- Extra-glandular manifestations include:
  - Joint involvement
  - Lung disease
  - Renal disease
  - Peripheral neuropathy
  - Gastrointestinal complaints
  - Autoimmune thyroid disorders.
- About 2–5% of people with SS develop lymphomas.

Clinical signs

Dry mouth is often the most characteristic feature in Sjögren syndrome (Figure 8.7).

Salivary gland swelling may appear (Figure 8.8), shown here in the sub-mandibular salivary glands.

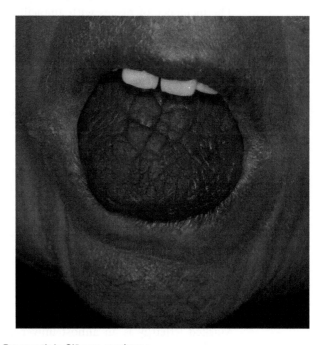

Figure 8.7   Dry mouth in Sjögren syndrome

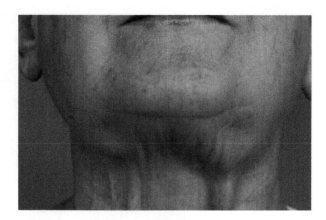

Figure 8.8 Swelling of the submandibular salivary glands

Table 8.2 Sjögren syndrome EU/USA consensus criteria: Vitali et al. 2002

Feature	
Ocular symptoms	Dryness >3/12; sensation of grit; need to use teardrops
Oral symptoms	Dryness >3/12; salivary gland swelling; need for liquids to help swallowing
Ocular signs	Schirmer <5 mm/5 min; positive Rose Bengal/Lissamine Green staining
Histology*	Labial salivary gland Bx
Objective salivary gland involvement	Flow rate <1.5 mL/15 min; sialography; scintigraphy
Autoantibodies*	SS-A [anti-Ro] and/or SS-B [anti-La] positive

Diagnosis: 4 out of 6 features with at least one of those marked '*' positive.

Diagnosis

- Classification criteria developed and revised by the American–European Consensus Group are widely accepted for the diagnosis of Sjögren syndrome (Table 8.2).
- Investigations may include:
  - Salivary flow rates: reduced (unstimulated whole saliva flow rate <1.5 mL/min)
  - Schirmer 1 test for tear flow rate: reduced (<5 mm in 5 minutes)
  - Serum autoantibodies (especially antibodies to the extractable nuclear antigens SS-A [Ro: Robair] and SS-B [La: Lattimer]): common
  - Serum immunoglobulin levels: hypergammaglobulinaemia is a not infrequent finding, and in patients with primary SS is a risk factor for lymphoma development
  - Labial salivary gland biopsy: shows focal lymphocytic sialadenitis
  - Sialography: may show sialectasis
  - Scintigraphy: provides a functional assessment of salivary gland function
  - Ultrasound: reveals hypoechoic areas within affected salivary gland tissue (Figure 8.9).

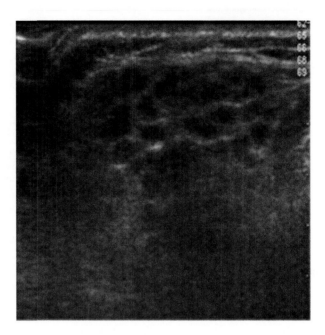

Figure 8.9   Ultrasound scan showing multiple hypoechoic areas within a parotid salivary gland in a patient with Sjögren syndrome (Courtesy, Mr PGJ Rout)

Management

- Management is symptomatic:
  - Dry mouth may be helped by sipping water or sugar-free drinks, sucking ice or using a salivary substitute or local sialogogue
  - Systemic sialogogues (muscarinic agonists) such as pilocarpine or cevimeline.
- Preventive dental care is important, embracing good oral hygiene practices and topical fluoride applications.
- There is interest in the potential for anti-B-cell therapy (e.g. rituximab).

Oral health care relevance

- Effects from persistent xerostomia, which can include:
  - Pain: from mucosal atrophy and candidosis
  - Disturbed oral function:
    - Difficulty in speaking, swallowing, or managing dentures
    - Taste changes
  - Infections:
    - Accelerated caries, particularly of smooth surfaces
    - Candidosis
    - Ascending (bacterial) sialadenitis
- Swelling of the major salivary glands
- Non-Hodgkin B-cell lymphomas (MALT-omas: mucosal associated lymphoid tissue-lymphomas).

9

Mucocutaneous conditions

Allergy

Allergy is an abnormal immune response to an allergen (e.g. a protein) and is usually considered to refer to either a Type I (immediate) or Type IV (delayed) hypersensitivity reaction. The classification of hypersensitivity reactions is summarised in Table 9.1 and common allergens in Table 9.2.

Type I (immediate) hypersensitivity is responsible for asthma, atopic eczema, allergic rhinitis (hayfever) and anaphylaxis. When an allergic (atopic) person is exposed to an allergen for the first time, IgE is synthesised in large amounts by plasma cells and becomes bound to the surface of mast cells and basophils. When the individual is re-challenged by the same antigen it interacts with this membrane-bound IgE antibody, causing degranulation of the mast cells and

Table 9.1 The classification of hypersensitivity reactions

Type	Nature	Examples
I	Immediate type hypersensitivity Ig-E mediated via mast cell degranulation	Anaphylaxis Atopic disorders
II	Antibody-mediated against membrane surface antigens	Blood transfusion reactions
III	Immune complex-mediated. Soluble immune complexes deposited in tissues	Systemic lupus erythematosus
IV	Delayed type hypersensitivity Cell (T-lymphocyte)-mediated	Contact allergies

Table 9.2 Common allergens

Allergen source	Hypersensitivity type	Examples
Food products	I	Egg, milk, nuts, shellfish
Drugs	I, III	Aspirin, penicillins, sulfonamides
Environmental	I, IV	Animal hair, dust mite, pollen
Latex	IV, I (rare)	Condoms, dressings, elastic bands, gloves
Dental materials	IV	Amalgam alloy, gold, mercury, resin-based materials

basophils with release of histamine and other mediators of inflammation. There is thus an immediate reaction.

Type IV (delayed) hypersensitivity is seen in skin contact allergies (and in the pathogenesis of granulomatous inflammatory diseases such as tuberculosis, leprosy and syphilis). This type of hypersensitivity is mediated by sensitised T-lymphocytes, which release cytokines that attract macrophages to the site of exposure. There is thus a delayed reaction appearing more than 24 hours after exposure to the allergen.

Latex allergy is a significant allergy in health care. It affects approximately 1% of the general population and is most often a contact allergy (Type IV delayed hypersensitivity) response, though a few patients display a Type I immediate hypersensitivity reaction. Latex allergy is an important occupational problem for health care workers where repeated rubber glove use, especially with abrasive hand-washing, increases the risk of sensitisation. Latex allergies are also common in patients frequently exposed to medical gloves during care and in individuals with long-term indwelling urinary latex catheters.

Latex is found in many items in the home and working environment including hospital clinics, wards and operating theatres. Latex exposure may occur via the skin, mucous membranes or bronchial tree with inhalation of latex glove powder. Due to allergen cross-reactivity, patients with a latex allergy may also react to certain foods (e.g. avocado, banana, chestnut and kiwi).

Clinical features

The clinical manifestations of an allergic reaction depend upon the nature of the allergic response, the antigenic challenge and the individual's 'allergic predisposition'.

Early symptoms and signs of a Type I (immediate) hypersensitivity reaction typically appear within a few minutes to an hour, and include: itching, breathlessness and urticaria. As the reaction progresses bronchospasm, hypotension and angio-oedema of the face and laryngopharynx may result in life-threatening anaphylactic shock.

Contact allergy (Type IV delayed hypersensitivity) appears over 24 hours or more and is characterised by local inflammation at the site of contact with the allergen (skin or mucous membrane). Physical factors (thermal stimuli, sunlight, water, pressure on the skin) may also result in the release of histamine in some susceptible individuals and cause similar features.

Clinical signs

Dermatitis on the hands in latex allergy is common in health care workers (Figure 9.1). Other allergies typically present as rashes, and often arise from exposure to drugs (Figure 9.2).

Diagnosis

Diagnosis of allergy is based on:

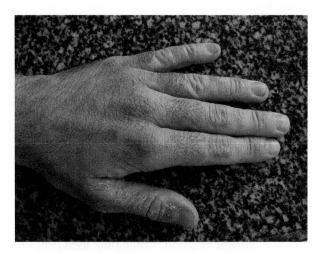

Figure 9.1   Dermatitis due to latex allergy

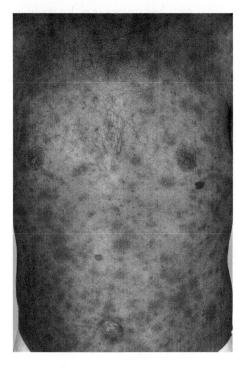

Figure 9.2   Rash due to a drug allergy

- Clinical history and presentation including often a family history of allergy
- IgE radioallergosorbent testing (RAST) for allergies considered to be Type I in nature. False positive results are not uncommon
- Serum mast cell tryptase estimation in suspected Type I reactions
- Skin-prick testing: identifies IgE sensitivity to common allergens allowing the diagnosis or exclusion of atopic disease
- Serum IgE levels: an alternative to skin-prick testing

- Patch testing to identify contact allergens using a battery of test allergens
- Elimination diet: used to identify food allergens.

Management

Allergies are best managed by allergen avoidance:

- House dust mite: mite-proof bed linen and wooden floors
- Pets: avoid or exclude
- Pollens: windows should be kept shut and grassy spaces avoided
- Food products: elimination diet
- Drugs: avoid. Accurately document drug allergies in medical notes. Medi-alert bracelets detailing an individual's allergies are also available.

Medical therapy may be indicated depending on the nature and severity of the allergic reaction. Commonly used drugs include:

- Mast cell stabilisers (e.g. sodium cromoglicate)
- Anti-histamines (e.g. loratadine, mizolastine, desloratadine): relieve itching and oedema
- Bronchodilators: management of bronchospasm
- Corticosteroids
- Adrenaline (epinephrine): management of anaphylaxis. Patients at risk of anaphylaxis should carry an Epi-pen (syringe of epinephrine) for self-administration.

Individuals with a complex history of allergy should be referred to a specialist allergy clinic for careful assessment and management.

Oral health care relevance

- Atopic patients (those with a history of asthma, eczema or hayfever) are more likely to be allergic to drugs such as penicillins.
- Angio-oedema with oedema of face, lips, tongue and neck may be a feature of an acute anaphylactic reaction.
- Allergic responses to drugs may manifest orofacially: e.g. angio-oedema associated with angiotensin converting enzyme inhibitors.
- Recurrent aphthous ulceration may occasionally be associated with dietary allergens (e.g. fish, nuts, eggs, chocolate) and a small number of patients respond to the appropriate exclusion diets. The precise mechanisms involved are uncertain.
- Some cases of orofacial granulomatosis are related to hypersensitivity reactions to dietary allergens, in particular, sodium benzoate preservatives and cinnamonaldehyde.
- Erythema migrans is believed to be more common in atopic individuals.
- Contact sensitivity reactions to dental materials can occur intra-orally (e.g. to nickel in susceptible patients).
- Anti-histamines can cause xerostomia.
- Drugs may interact with anti-histamines:
  - Imidazole and triazole anti-fungals inhibit mizolastine metabolism
  - Erythromycin inhibits mizolastine metabolism

- Erythromycin may increase the plasma concentration of loratadine
- Anti-retroviral drugs may increase the plasma concentration of various anti-histamines (e.g. chlorphenamine maleate, loratadine).

Lichen planus

Lichen planus is a common skin and mucosal disease associated with a dense reactive T-lymphocyte infiltrate beneath affected epithelia. Although the provoking antigen is unidentified, lesions clinically and histologically similar or identical to lichen planus (lichenoid lesions) can be related to:

- Dental restorations, particularly amalgam
- Drugs, particularly non-steroidal anti-inflammatory agents
- Chemicals, particularly photographic developing solutions
- Graft-versus-host disease
- Chronic liver disease
- Virus infections: hepatitis C or HIV.

Clinical features

- Skin lesions are usually small polygonal, purplish or violaceous, itchy papules with a lacy network of white striae (Wickham striae) particularly affecting the flexor surfaces of the wrists (Figure 9.3).
- Mouth, genitals, nails or hair may be affected in addition or in isolation.

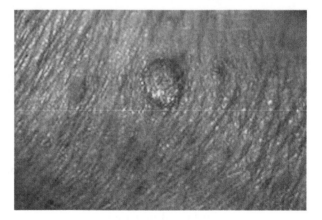

Figure 9.3   Itchy papules with Wickham striae

Clinical signs

- Lichenoid white bilateral lesions on buccal mucosae or the tongue (Figure 9.4).

Diagnosis

- A drug history should exclude possible reactions.
- Biopsy may be indicated.

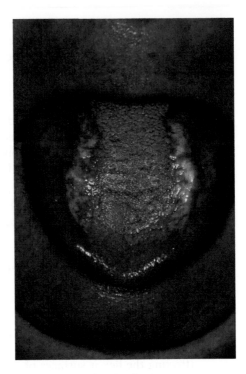

Figure 9.4   Lichenoid white bilateral lesions on the tongue as a consequence of indometacin medication

Management

- Topical corticosteroids to control symptomatic lichen planus.
- Severe lichen planus sometimes responds only to systemic corticosteroids.

Oral health care relevance

- Mouth lesions include white striae, papules, plaques or red atrophic areas, and/or erosions or ulcers.
- Oral lesions are characteristically bilateral and affect particularly the posterior buccal mucosae.
- Gingival lesions, if present, are usually atrophic and red ('desquamative gingivitis').
- It is important to consider the possibility of lichenoid reactions to drugs. A detailed drug history is important in management (Table 9.3).
- Dental amalgam may also provoke lichenoid reactions in some patients.
- Lichen planus has a small malignant potential: approximately 1% of cases may develop carcinoma after 10 years. Erosive and plaque like lesions should be particularly monitored in this respect. Six-monthly review intervals would seem appropriate but if there is histological evidence of dysplasia, closer follow-up intervals might be prudent.

Table 9.3   Some drugs capable of inducing oral lichenoid reactions

More frequently prescribed drugs	Less frequently prescribed drugs
Non-steroidal anti inflammatory drugs	Allopurinol
Anti-hypertensive agents:	Gold
<ul><li>Beta blockers</li><li>Thiazide diuretics</li><li>Calcium channel blockers</li><li>Angiotensin converting enzyme inhibitors</li></ul>	
Oral hypoglycaemic agents	Penicillamine
<ul><li>Sulphonylureas</li><li>Metformin</li></ul>	
Tricyclic antidepressants	Antimalarials Streptomycin

Behçet disease

Immune complexes (antigen–antibody complexes) underlie certain diseases, by inducing complement activation and vasculitis. Behçet disease and erythema multiforme are important in this respect.

Behçet disease is a clinical triad of oral and genital ulceration, and uveitis.

It mainly affects young adult males with 'Silk Road' bloodlines, particularly from Turkey, Central Asia, Japan and Korea. There is an association with *HLA-B5* and *HLA-B5101*.

Clinical features

- Behçet disease is a potentially lethal, multisystem disease but oral ulceration similar to aphthae is the most constant feature.
- Ocular, cutaneous and genital lesions are also common.

Clinical signs

Erythema nodosum (Figure 9.5) – tender red/purple nodules commonly occurring over the lower limbs and healing with a bruised appearance – may be associated with Behçet disease as well as a variety of other causes including sarcoidosis, inflammatory bowel disease and certain drugs such as sulfonamides.

Diagnosis

- Behçet disease is diagnosed mainly on clinical grounds but *HLA-B5101* and pathergy (a skin prick test performed during active Behçet symptoms) are helpful.

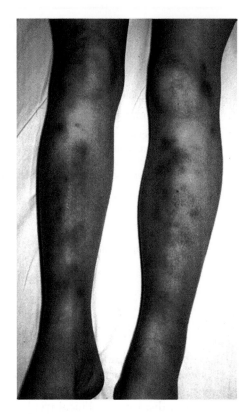

Figure 9.5   Erythema nodosum

- The International Study Group criteria for classification of Behçet Disease are:
  - Recurrent mouth ulceration
  - Plus any two of the following:
    - Recurrent genital ulceration
    - Eye inflammation
    - Skin lesions
    - A positive pathergy test.

Management

- Medical and ophthalmological help should be obtained.
- Treatments include mainly immunosuppressive drugs.

Oral health care relevance

- Oral lesions resemble, and can be managed like, common aphthae.
- Intractable oral ulceration may be managed with colchicine, or agents with anti-tumour necrosis factor-alpha (anti-TNF-alpha) activity such as thalidomide or infliximab.

- Patients may also be treated with immunosuppressive agents (e.g. ciclosporin), which will have dental implications (e.g. gingival overgrowth).
- It is important that the possibility of Behçet disease is not overlooked when managing patients apparently suffering recurrent aphthous stomatitis.

Erythema multiforme

Erythema multiforme primarily affects young males and is characterised by mucosal and/or cutaneous lesions, different rashes (hence the term 'multiforme') and is often recurrent.

Erythema multiforme is an uncommon disorder, which may be an immune complex disorder in which the antigens can be various microorganisms (e.g. mycoplasmas) or drugs (e.g. penicillins, aspirin, sulfonamides and carbamazepine). Herpes simplex virus appears to be responsible for most recurrent cases.

Clinical features

- Skin and ocular, genital or oral mucous membranes may be involved together or in isolation.
- The typical lesion is the skin target or iris lesion of concentric erythematous rings, affecting particularly the hands and feet.
- Typical oral features are widespread ulceration and swollen, crusted and blood-stained lips.
- Severe cases with multiple mucosal involvement and fever are termed Stevens–Johnson syndrome, or toxic epidermal necrolysis (TEN).

Clinical signs

Serosanguinous lesions on the lips (Figure 9.6) are almost pathognomonic of erythema multiforme but similar lesions may be seen in para-neoplastic

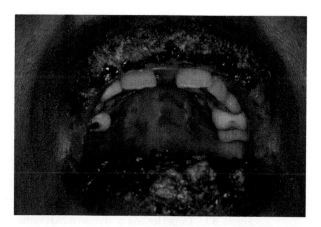

Figure 9.6 Serosanguinous lesions on the lips and mouth ulceration in erythema multiforme

pemphigus. Similarly, target or iris lesions on the skin (Figures 9.7 and 9.8) are very typical of erythema multiforme but again are not absolutely specific. Severe skin sloughing may be seen in drug-induced lesions of toxic epidermal necrolysis (Figure 9.9).

Diagnosis

- The diagnosis is usually on clinical grounds but biopsy may be indicated.

Management

- Oral lesions can be symptomatically managed.
- Severe disease may necessitate hospital admission as feeding may be difficult.

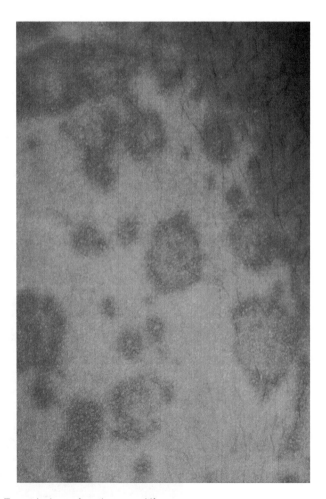

Figure 9.7   Target lesions of erythema multiforme

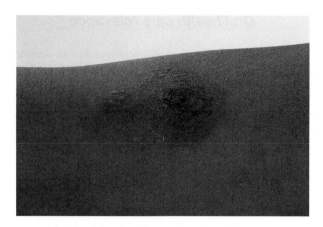

Figure 9.8 Target lesion of erythema multiforme

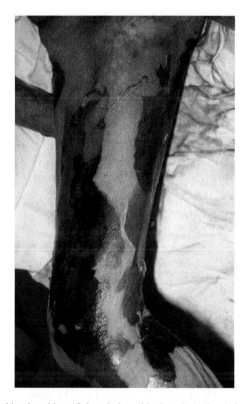

Figure 9.9 Severe skin sloughing of drug-induced lesions in toxic epidermal necrolysis

- Oral corticosteroids (prednisolone) may be helpful in managing the acute phase, but do not prevent recurrence.
- Anti-virals are indicated for prophylaxis of recurrent erythema multiforme.
- Antibiotics may help if mycoplasma infection is involved.
- Identifiable triggers should be avoided.

Oral health care relevance

- Orofacial manifestations are as described above.
- It is important to differentiate this condition from primary herpetic gingivostomatitis:
  - A previous attack suggests erythema multiforme
  - A prodrome occurs in herpes but not usually in erythema multiforme
  - Target lesions are almost pathognomonic of erythema multiforme
  - There is usually less constitutional upset, pyrexia and lymphadenopathy in erythema multiforme.
- In major erythema multiforme, there is widespread cutaneous, mucosal and visceral involvement and the condition may be life threatening.
- Recently, the risk of carbamazepine-induced Stevens–Johnson syndrome has been associated with the *HLA-B1502* allele in Han Chinese, Hong Kong Chinese and Thai populations.

Pemphigoid

Damage to proteins that bind epithelial cells one to another, or to the epithelial basement membrane, can lead to blistering diseases of the skin and/or mucosae; these are termed vesiculobullous disorders. Most are acquired autoimmune disorders, and pemphigoid and pemphigus are the most important.

Mucous membrane pemphigoid is a group of sub-epithelial autoimmune blistering diseases with autoantibodies directed to different epithelial basement membrane proteins, causing loss of attachment of the epithelium to the connective tissue and blister formation.

Clinical features

- Intact oral mucosal vesicles or bullae are frequently seen.
- Rupture of the vesicles or bullae results in painful, shallow, ragged areas of ulceration, often involving the distal hard palate and soft palate.
- The gingivae are often affected by 'desquamative gingivitis'.
- Scarring is a serious potential complication in eyes, larynx, oesophagus or genitalia.

Clinical signs

Ocular involvement may be seen in mucous membrane pemphigoid (Figure 9.10) and can seriously compromise sight. The feature shown is an entropion – an in-turning of the eyelid due to scarring of the conjunctiva and subsequent scar contraction. Skin blisters are uncommon in oral pemphigoid (Figure 9.11).

Diagnosis

- Blistering conditions such as mucous membrane pemphigoid, pemphigus,

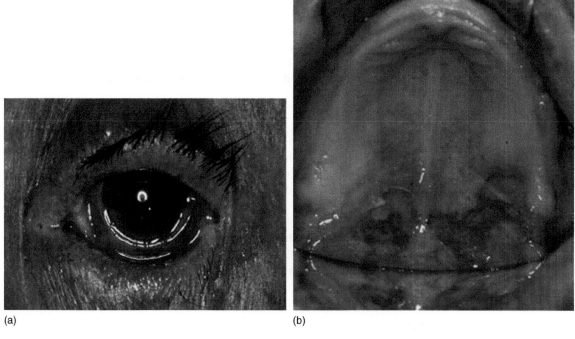

(a)   (b)

Figure 9.10 Mucous membrane pemphigoid: (a) entropion and (b) oral ulceration

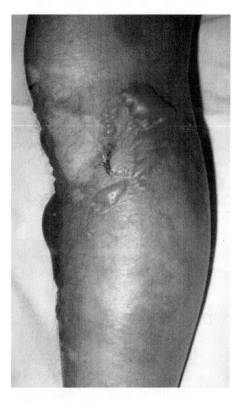

Figure 9.11 Skin blisters in pemphigoid

angina bullosa haemorrhagica, linear IgA disease and dermatitis herpeti-formis can be difficult to differentiate clinically.
- Stroking the skin or mucosa with a finger may induce vesicle formation in an apparently unaffected area or cause a bulla to extend (Nikolsky sign).
- The diagnosis must be confirmed by biopsy and immunostaining (direct immunofluorescence) and indirect immunofluorescence on a serum sample.

Management

- An ophthalmological referral is essential to exclude insidious eye disease.
- Oral lesions can often be controlled by topical or oral corticosteroids or dapsone, dependent on disease severity and distribution.

Oral health care relevance

- Orofacial manifestations are as described above.

Pemphigus

Pemphigus is an uncommon potentially fatal autoimmune reaction against proteins in stratified squamous epithelium. Autoantibodies in the common form (pemphigus vulgaris) are directed against desmoglein-3 of intercellular attachments (desmosomes) of epithelial cells.

Clinical features

- Pemphigus is characterised by widespread intra-epithelial vesicles and bullae, frequently first appearing in the mouth.
- The blisters rupture and, in the absence of treatment, pemphigus is usually fatal.

Clinical signs

Flaccid blisters appear mainly in traumatised areas (Figure 9.12) and break to form scabs on the skin (Figure 9.13) and erosions in the mouth (Figure 9.14).

Diagnosis

- Stroking the skin or mucosa with a finger may induce vesicle formation in an apparently unaffected area or cause a bulla to extend (Nikolsky sign).
- Diagnosis must be confirmed by biopsy and immunostaining.

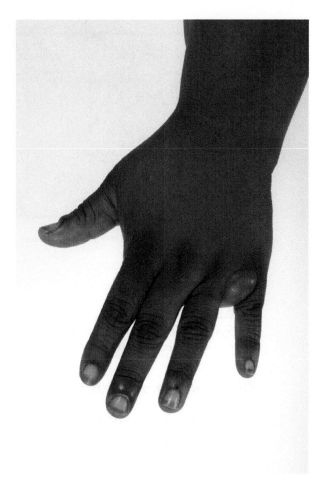

Figure 9.12   Flaccid blisters of pemphigus

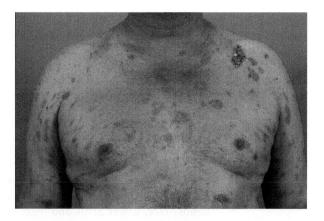

Figure 9.13   Scabs on the skin where blisters have burst

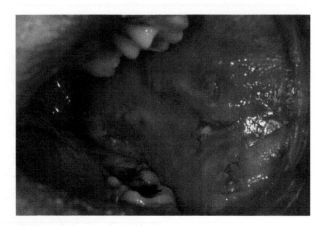

Figure 9.14   Erosions in the mouth where blisters have burst

Management

- Patients should be under the care of a physician.
- Systemic corticosteroids plus a steroid-sparing agent such as azathioprine, or mycophenolate are typically needed.

Oral health care relevance

- Oral mucosal involvement is common and may be the initial presenting sign often many months ahead of other sites.
- Bullae are very fragile and flaccid rupturing within a few hours. The resultant ulcerations are often very irregular and slit-like in appearance.
- Desquamative gingivitis is common.

Scleroderma

Scleroderma, means hard skin (from the Greek 'skleros' = hard, 'derma' = skin). It is associated with anti-nuclear antibodies directed against topoisomerase or centromeres and results in fibroblasts producing excess collagen.

Clinical features

Scleroderma can be localised to skin and related tissues, or systemic.

- Localised scleroderma: never progresses to a systemic form.
- Systemic sclerosis (scleroderma): involves deeper tissues (blood vessels and major organs) also, and may manifest as:
  - Limited scleroderma: affects the skin only in certain areas: the fingers, hands, face, lower arms and legs; and many people have CREST:
    - Calcinosis: calcium deposits typically on the fingers, hands, face and trunk

- Raynaud phenomenon
- OEsophageal dysfunction
- Sclerodactyly: thick and tight skin on the fingers
- Telangiectasias.
- Diffuse scleroderma: affects hands, face, upper arms, upper legs, chest and stomach in a symmetrical fashion, and one third develop renal, pulmonary, gastrointestinal or cardiac disease.

Clinical signs

Facial movement is restricted (Mona Lisa face), the nose may appear 'pinched', mouth opening becomes progressively limited (fish-mouth; Figure 9.15) and telangiectasia may be seen on the lips and intraorally, especially on the tongue.

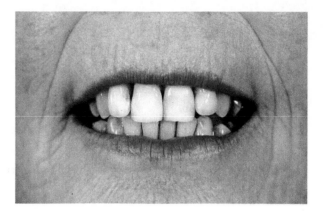

Figure 9.15 Mouth opening becomes limited in scleroderma

The orofacial tissues show multiple telangiectasia, whilst the hands show sclerodactyly and calcinosis (small subcutaneous calcific deposits) (Figure 9.16). These features together with the history are strongly suggestive of CREST syndrome. Widening of the periodontal space is a characteristic, if uncommon, feature (Figure 9.17). Tooth mobility, however, is not increased.

Diagnosis

- Limited systemic sclerosis: serum anti-centromere antibodies are found in up to 90% of patients.
- Diffuse systemic sclerosis: serum anti-topoisomerase-1 antibodies are found in up to 40% of patients.

Management

- There is no specific treatment but newer therapies under trial include anti-transforming growth factor-beta (anti-TGF-beta), stem cell transplantation and endothelin antagonists.

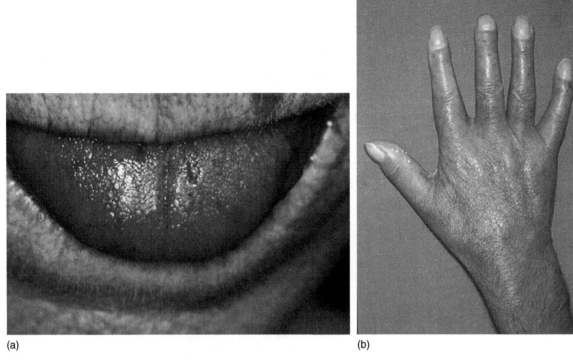

(a)　　　　　　　　　　　　　　　　　　　　　　　(b)

Figure 9.16　(a) Multiple telangiectasia of the orofacial tissues and (b) sclerodactyly and calcinosis of the hands in scleroderma

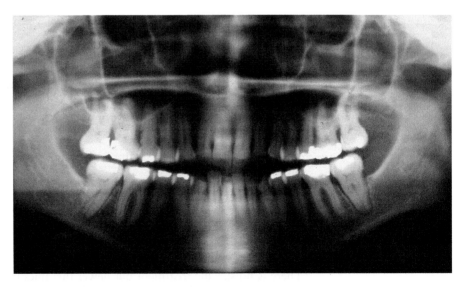

Figure 9.17　Widening of the periodontal space in scleroderma

Oral health care relevance

- Most patients have orofacial manifestations (see p. 141) and these may be the presenting signs in 30% of affected individuals:
  - The tongue may become stiff (chicken tongue)
  - Bony changes including resorption of the mandibular angle and coronoid process may occur.
- Secondary Sjögren syndrome develops in a significant number of cases.

Systemic lupus erythematosus

Systemic lupus erythematosus (SLE) is a potentially lethal disease with autoantibodies to DNA, which cause vasculitis and multisystem involvement.

Clinical features

- Systemic lupus erythematosus can cause a wide variety of clinical pictures depending on the organs predominantly affected.
- Classically, there are fevers, malaise, anaemia, joint pains and a rash.
- Renal involvement is common: proteinuria and haematuria, often associated with hypertension, are seen.

Clinical signs

The 'butterfly rash' is typical of SLE (Figure 9.18): a similar appearance is seen in patients with mitral stenosis (Figure 1.9, p. 15). Raynaud phenomenon is common.

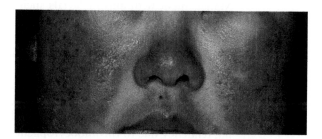

Figure 9.18　The 'butterfly rash' is typical of systemic lupus erythematosus

Oral manifestations include ulceration, dry mouth as a consequence of Sjögren syndrome (perhaps in 30–50% patients) and lesions that mimic lichen planus. Lichenoid reactions may also arise as a consequence of the patient's medication.

Diagnosis

- The American College of Rheumatology diagnostic criteria for SLE are based on the presence of at least 4 of the following:
  - Malar rash
  - Discoid rash
  - Photosensitivity
  - Mouth ulcers
  - Arthritis
  - Serositis (pleuritis or pericarditis)
  - Renal disorder
  - Neurological disorder
  - Haematologic disorder
  - Immunologic disorder.
- Systemic lupus erythematosus is confirmed by serology (e.g. anti-nuclear antibodies (ANA) especially anti-double-stranded DNA or anti-Sm antibody), and biopsy of skin or kidney using immunofluorescent staining.

Management

- Corticosteroids are useful to control early acute, and potentially lethal complications such as renal involvement.
- Otherwise, most patients do well with non-steroidal anti-inflammatory drugs (NSAIDs) or anti-malarials.

Oral health care relevance

- Oral lesions include erythematous areas, erosions, ulcers or white lesions that mimic lichen planus.
- Sjögren syndrome is associated in up to 30% or more of cases.
- Management with anti-malarials such as hydroxychloroquine may predispose susceptible patients to lichenoid reactions.
- Management with corticosteroids may predispose patients to Addisonian shock, and steroid boosting will be desirable in some of these patients who undergo invasive dental procedures.
- Other immunosuppressive agents used in the management of SLE may also influence the dental management of these patients.
- Patients with SLE may have endocardial damage, renal disease, and a bleeding tendency due to thrombocytopaenia, which may impact on the delivery of dental treatment.
- Some patients with SLE have an associated anti-phospholipid syndrome, and as a result may be taking anticoagulants such as warfarin.

10 Infectious diseases

HIV infection and AIDS

The human immunodeficiency virus (HIV) is a retrovirus that infects mainly CD4+ cells, especially helper T-lymphocytes and brain microglia. It damages these over months and years, to eventually cause AIDS (acquired immune deficiency syndrome) with a predisposition particularly to infections with viruses, fungi and mycobacteria. Several subtypes of HIV including drug resistant forms have been identified.

HIV is transmitted by:

- Sexual intercourse: saliva, semen and blood may contain HIV
- Contaminated blood, blood products and donated organs
- Contaminated needles: intravenous drug users and needlestick injuries in health care workers
- Vertical transmission (mother to child): may occur *in utero*, during childbirth or via breast milk.

There is no reliable evidence for transmission of HIV by non-sexual social contact or by potential insect vectors such as mosquitoes.

HIV has spread to create a global pandemic: southern Africa and Asia bear the greatest burden of disease.

Clinical features

HIV infection may be staged according to its clinical features (Table 10.1).

Table 10.1   The classification of HIV infection

CDC stage	Presentation
1	Primary seroconversion illness
2	Asymptomatic disease
3	Persistent generalised lymphadenopathy (PGL)
4a	AIDS related complex (ARC)
4b–d	AIDS (AIDS defining illness)

CDC: Centers for Disease Control and Prevention, Atlanta, Georgia, USA.

After primary infection with HIV an acute viraemia causes widespread viral dissemination and, in about one third, a glandular fever type syndrome with malaise, fever, lymphadenopathy and mouth ulcers. Serum antibodies to HIV appear within 6 weeks to 6 months of infection (seroconversion).

An asymptomatic period of variable length generally follows seroconversion but, as HIV infection of CD4+ cells leads to lymphopaenia and a reduced CD4+ to CD8+ T-lymphocyte ratio, severe cell-mediated immunodeficiency and symptoms of disease subsequently develop (HIV-related disease).

AIDS is defined as a CD4 count of <200/mm^3 of blood, in a patient infected with HIV, and develops within 5 years of infection in about 20% of HIV-positive individuals. AIDS develops in the others over the next 5 to 10 years.

Common manifestations of HIV /AIDS include:

- Infections: with opportunistic pathogens, especially fungi, viruses, mycobacteria and parasites (e.g. candidosis, herpesvirus infections, tuberculosis, toxoplasmosis, *Pneumocystis carinii* [*jiroveci*] pneumonia)
- Malignant neoplasms (Kaposi sarcoma, non-Hodgkin lymphoma, cervical cancer): which often have a viral aetiology
- Neurological disease (AIDS-related dementia)
- Autoimmune disorders (autoimmune thrombocytopaenia)
- Weight loss and wasting – 'slim disease'.

Clinical signs

Viral infections such as herpesvirus infections (herpes labialis, varicella zoster or shingles, and hairy leukoplakia) and other viruses such as human papillomavirus and molluscum contagiosum (Figure 10.1), and fungal infections such as candidosis (Figure 10.2) are common. Oral candidosis in HIV/AIDS is common and may present with white or red, or mixed lesions (Figure 10.2 shows predominantly red palatal lesions, and white lesions mainly in the distal buccal sulcus).

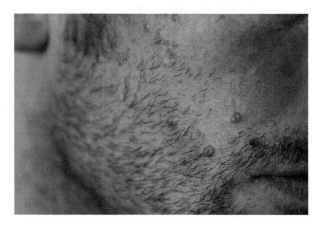

Figure 10.1 Molluscum contagiosum

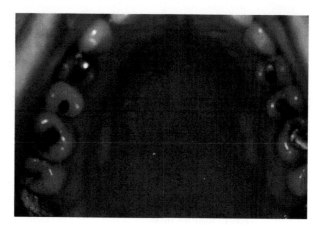

Figure 10.2 Candidosis

Hypersensitivity to some drugs may also occur in certain individuals. Adverse effects from anti-retroviral drugs vary by drug, by ethnicity and by individual, as well as by interaction with other drugs, including alcohol. Adverse effects can include pigmentation from zidovudine (Figure 10.3) but they are wide ranging and can include oral effects such as dry mouth and ulceration.

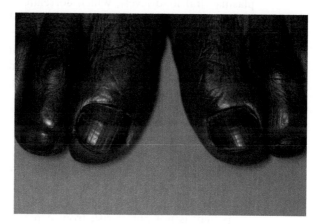

Figure 10.3 Pigmentation due to treatment with zidovudine

Treatment with anti-retroviral drugs may also result in rapid suppression of HIV and partial restoration of the immune system, sometimes producing a dangerous hypersensitivity reaction termed the immune reconstitution inflammatory syndrome (IRIS), which can manifest with severe zoster or papillomavirus infections and other sequelae.

Diagnosis

The diagnosis of HIV infection is based upon the following:

- A history of potential exposure to HIV
- The pattern of clinical presentation
- Full blood count (lymphopaenia)
- Low T-CD4 count and reduced CD4:CD8 ratio
- Serum antibodies to HIV detected by enzyme-linked immunosorbent assay (ELISA) or agglutination screening tests and a supplemental confirmatory test such as Western immunoblotting.

Management

The mortality rate from AIDS is virtually 100%, although anti-retroviral drugs can significantly impede the progress of HIV infection. Anti-retroviral therapy (ART) can include:

- Nucleoside analogues (e.g. zidovudine)
- Non-nucleoside reverse transcriptase inhibitors (e.g. nevirapine)
- Protease inhibitors (e.g. indinavir).

Treatment with a combination of these drugs is termed highly active anti-retroviral therapy (HAART). Adverse effects are common and adherence to therapy is important to avoid the development of drug-resistant variants. Patients on anti-retroviral therapy are monitored by regular CD4 counts and plasma viral load levels, which correlate well with clinical response. Patients with low CD4 counts are given anti-microbials as prophylaxis against opportunistic infections. There is still no effective treatment for the underlying immune defect. Individuals should also be offered psychological support to help them come to terms with their illness and should be educated on measures necessary to prevent further cross-infection.

Oral health care relevance

- It is important to ascertain the severity of the condition with the patient's genitourinary medicine consultant, who will be able to provide details of the patient's medication and any specific issues relating to dental care.
- Strict asepsis is most important to ensure that the immunocompromised patient is not put at risk from dental treatment, particularly if their CD4 count is low. Patients with full blown AIDS who are markedly immunocompromised may be best managed in specialist units. Otherwise, the need for strict infection control procedures is as paramount as it is for any patient. The patient may also be infected with hepatitis B or C, and the risk of transmitting these infections to other patients is much greater than that for HIV.
- The medical management of HIV disease is complex, requiring combination therapy with reverse transcriptase inhibitors, protease inhibitors and other agents. Some anti-retroviral drugs may interact with a number of drugs commonly used in dentistry e.g. ritonavir increases plasma concentration of carbamazepine. Its concurrent administration with midazolam must be avoided as it may precipitate excessive sedation and possibly respiratory

depression. Anti-retroviral drugs may produce oral manifestations, e.g. xerostomia (nelfinavir, ritonavir), mucosal pigmentation (zidovudine).

- The orofacial manifestations of HIV/AIDS are protean and beyond the scope of this book but some of the more common lesions that may be associated with HIV/AIDS infection include:
  - Cervical lymphadenopathy
  - Infections:
    - Candidosis (often thrush or erythematous), may be a presenting feature of HIV infection
    - Herpes infections, including simplex, zoster, cytomegalovirus and Epstein–Barr virus (hairy leukoplakia related to EBV)
    - Periodontal disease, including necrotising gingivitis/stomatitis
  - Neoplasms:
    - Kaposi sarcoma (caused by human herpesvirus 8)
    - Lymphomas (often caused by EBV)
  - Salivary gland swelling and xerostomia.

In the event of a member of the dental team sustaining a sharps injury from a patient with HIV/AIDS they should wash the injured area copiously as for other sharps injuries and seek immediate counselling for post-exposure prophylaxis (PEP: a short course of anti-retrovirals, aimed at eradicating any virus that may have been transmitted via the injury). Prophylaxis, if appropriate, needs to be administered as soon as possible after injury, ideally within 1 hour, and at most within 72 hours. It can be accessed via accident and emergency departments or via occupational health departments dependent on circumstances.

Herpesviruses: Herpes simplex virus (HSV: human herpesviruses type 1 and 2) infections

Herpesviruses are DNA viruses, which are ubiquitous, and can be spread by saliva or other body fluids. After primary infection, these viruses remain latent, often in neurones. Reactivation (often in immunocompromising states) may lead to viral shedding and disease.

Herpes simplex virus (HSV) occurs in two types: type 1 and type 2.

Clinical features

- Type 1 HSV:
  - Typically causes primary oral infection with acute gingivostomatitis
  - May cause primary anogenital infection.
- Type 2 HSV:
  - Typically causes anogenital infections
  - May cause oral or oropharyngeal infections.
- HSV thereafter remains latent in the sensory ganglia but if reactivated may cause recurrent infections.

- Recurrent infections typically affect the mucocutaneous junctions and are often precipitated by factors such as exposure to systemic infections, sunlight, trauma, stress, menstruation or immune incompetence.

Clinical signs

Type I HSV is usually responsible for primary and recurrent (Figure 10.4) oral and peri-oral herpes, although type 2 infection (which usually causes genital infection) can sometimes be isolated. Recurrent attacks may be seen in 30% of cases, and there may be bacterial super-infection – typically staphylococcal.

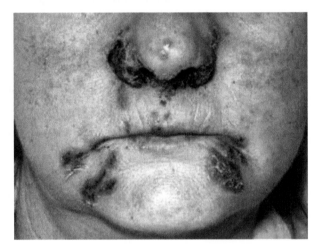

Figure 10.4   Herpes simplex virus type 1 infection resulting in oral and peri-oral herpes

Diagnosis

- Diagnosis is typically clinical.

Management

- Aciclovir, famciclovir or other anti-virals are effective in primary infections, but many patients present with disease too far advanced to benefit. Anti-virals are essential to control infection in immunocompromised patients.
- Supportive care includes adequate fluid intake, anti-pyretics and analgesics (usually paracetamol) and good oral hygiene.
- Recurrent herpes labialis infections respond to penciclovir or aciclovir cream if applied at the onset of the infection.

Oral health care relevance

- Generally an infection of young children, usually involving type 1 HSV. The natural history is changing with an increased prevalence in young, particularly male, adults. Additionally there is an increase in oral HSV-2 infections (the serotype more commonly involved in anogenital herpes infections).

- The primary infection is often subclinical, but typical clinical features of primary herpetic gingivostomatitis include:
  - Prodrome: non-specific malaise similar to influenza occurs 2–4 days prior to oral manifestations becoming apparent
  - Oral lesions start as blisters which often go unnoticed as they are painless
  - The blisters rupture to form shallow ulcers, which coalesce into serpiginous erosions on the palate, tongue, floor of mouth and buccal mucosa
  - The gingivae become sore, swollen and inflamed
  - Lip erosions become crusted with a bloody fibrinopurulent exudate
  - Patients are pyrexial, exhibit regional lymphadenopathy and feel generally unwell.
- The infection is usually self-limiting within 10–14 days, although more generalised and serious infection may occur in immunocompromised patients or those with eczema.
- Differential diagnosis includes:
  - Erythema multiforme
  - Herpetiform aphthae
  - Leukaemias
  - Coxsackie virus infections.
- Diagnosis is usually made on clinical features, but smears to identify cytopathic changes – such as ballooning degeneration of epithelial cells, intranuclear inclusion bodies and mulberry nuclei – can be helpful, as may identification of viral DNA or the virus itself by immunostaining or electron microscopy.
- Once infected, HSV is not eliminated from the body but remains in the trigeminal ganglion. Recurrent infections in those susceptible (approximately 30% of patients) manifest as cold sores, which may be precipitated by sunlight, stress, other infections and trauma.
- Recurrent infections suggest a cell-mediated immune defect.
- The patient should be warned of the potential to transmit the infection to the eye and therefore avoid finger contact with the herpetic lesions and rubbing their eyes. Equally, finger contact with the lesions can transmit the infection to the nail-beds (herpetic whitlow) of the patient or indeed the dental care professional if for some reason they are not gloved.
- Treatment of primary herpetic gingivostomatitis:
  - Supportive measures: fluids, bed rest and topical local anaesthetics
  - The patient may need to be admitted to hospital if unable to swallow fluids
  - Antibacterial agents, e.g. chlorhexidine mouthwash, to reduce secondary infection
  - Systemic aciclovir: to be effective should be started as soon as possible in the course of the infection
  - Topical 5% aciclovir or 1% penciclovir creams can be helpful in treating recurrent herpes labialis (herpetic cold sores), provided the antiviral is applied early. The patient must be instructed on how to apply

the preparation to ensure they do not transmit the infection to their nail-beds.

Herpesviruses: Varicella-zoster virus (VZV: human herpesvirus type 3) infections

Varicella (chickenpox) is a highly contagious disease mainly of children, caused by the varicella-zoster virus (VZV), spread readily by droplets.

Thereafter, VZV remains latent within dorsal root ganglia and, if reactivated, as can happen in older or immunocompromised people, can lead to shingles (zoster) – a painful unilateral rash. Herpes zoster may affect any age group, but it is much more common in adults over 60 years old, in children who had chickenpox before the age of one year and in individuals whose immune system is compromised.

Clinical features

- Zoster involves a sensory dermatome, usually in the thoracic region.
- There is pain and a rash in the dermatome.
- Trigeminal ophthalmic zoster may cause facial rash and pain and ulcerate the cornea.
- Trigeminal maxillary or mandibular zoster may cause a facial rash and pain (sometimes simulating toothache) and oral ulceration.

Clinical signs

Herpes zoster, an acute localised recurrence with varicella-zoster virus, causes an acute blistering rash (Figure 10.5) termed 'shingles', which typically follows the path of the trigeminal nerve in the face and is associated with mucosal ulceration and intense pain.

Shingles may be complicated by post-herpetic neuralgia – persistent pain in the area where the shingles occurred that may last from months to years following the initial episode. This pain can be severe enough to be incapacitating. Older people are at higher risk for this complication.

Diagnosis

- Diagnosis is clinical.

Management

- Patients with ophthalmic zoster should have an urgent ophthalmological opinion. Eye lesions may lead to permanent blindness if not treated with emergency medical care.
- Treatment of zoster is with aciclovir, valaciclovir or famciclovir

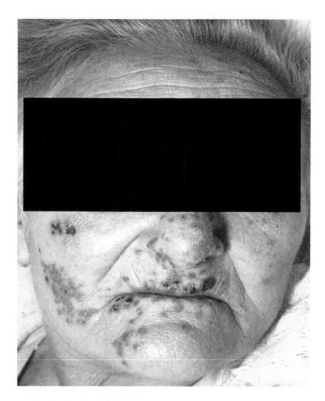

Figure 10.5   Herpes zoster (shingles)

Oral health care relevance

- Shingles in the young should raise the question about the immune status of the patient (e.g. lymphoma or possible HIV infection may be identified in approximately 10% of cases).
- Shingles produces pain and a vesicular rash over the dermatome supplied by the affected sensory nerve. The clinical features are typically unilateral although occasionally they may be bilateral. Vesiculation occurs on the facial skin and the corresponding oral mucosa.
- The pain may mimic toothache when the maxillary and/or mandibular divisions of the trigeminal nerve are involved. Pain usually predates the appearance of the rash and may be lancinating in character.
- Facial nerve geniculate ganglion involvement results in a lower motor neurone facial palsy with vesicles in the external auditory meatus, facial skin and around the ear and ear canal and in the pharynx, hearing loss and loss of taste in half of the tongue (Ramsay Hunt syndrome).
- Treatment with systemic anti-virals such as aciclovir 800 mg 5× daily for 7 days must be started early if it is to be effective.
- Post-herpetic neuralgia occurs in some 10% of patients following the acute attack. This responds poorly to analgesics and may be managed with tricyclic antidepressants such as amitriptyline or, if unsuccessful, gabapentin.

Herpesviruses: Epstein–Barr virus (EBV: human herpesvirus type 4) infections

Epstein–Barr virus (EBV) is transmitted mainly in saliva and causes infectious mononucleosis (IM: classic glandular fever), hairy leukoplakia, Burkitt and some other lymphomas and nasopharyngeal carcinoma.

Clinical features

● Infectious mononucleosis causes mainly lymphadenopathy, sore throat, fever and malaise, but is protean in its manifestations.

Clinical signs

Allergic reactions to ampicillin are common leading to a widespread rash (Figure 10.6).

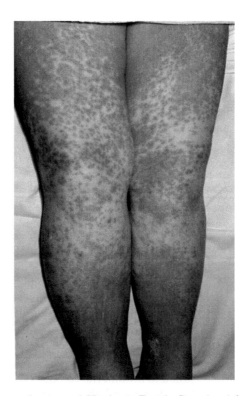

Figure 10.6   Allergic reaction to ampicillin due to Epstein–Barr virus infection

Diagnosis

Serological changes diagnostic of IM include heterophile antibodies (Paul–Bunnell test), which are transient, and EBV antibodies.

Management

There is no reliably effective specific treatment available for EBV infection, but the patient may benefit from bed rest.

Oral health care relevance

- Infectious mononucleosis may produce ulceration and inflammation in the mouth, particularly the oropharynx, in young adults. Additionally, petechial haemorrhages may present on the soft palate. The infection is often associated with marked regional lymphadenopathy, fever and malaise.
- Epstein–Barr virus is the aetiological agent in hairy leukoplakia. This may arise in immunocompromised individuals (e.g. in HIV disease and patients taking ciclosporin).

Epstein–Barr virus has also been suggested as a potential aetiological agent in Sjögren syndrome.

Tuberculosis

Tuberculosis (TB) is a major global health problem that affects approximately 1.5 billion people worldwide – one third of the world population. It is particularly widespread in developing countries and its incidence is increasing in Western countries (including the UK). Approximately 10% of cases are antibiotic resistant – multi-drug resistant (MDR) TB. Cases of extended drug resistant TB (XDR-TB), resistant to most drugs, have appeared mainly in HIV-infected patients.

Infection is most often due to *Mycobacterium tuberculosis* and is primarily a respiratory disease (pulmonary TB). It may also be caused by other atypical (non-tuberculous) mycobacteria such as *Mycobacterium avium* complex (MAC). Pulmonary TB is usually transmitted by infected sputum via droplet spread and the respiratory route.

Clinical features

Initial TB infection is usually subclinical: a primary lesion forms (usually pulmonary) and infection is confined to local lymph nodes – 'primary TB'. Active TB typically causes a chronic productive cough, haemoptysis, weight loss, night sweats and fever.

Reactivation or progression of primary TB may result in widespread haematogenous dissemination of mycobacteria throughout the body – 'miliary TB'. Multiple small lesions may affect the central nervous, cardiovascular, gastrointestinal and genitourinary systems. Clinical presentation is variable depending on the extent of spread and the organs involved.

Clinical signs

Cervical lymph node enlargement may be seen (Figure 10.7).

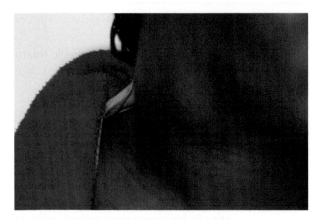

Figure 10.7   Cervical lymph node enlargement in tuberculosis

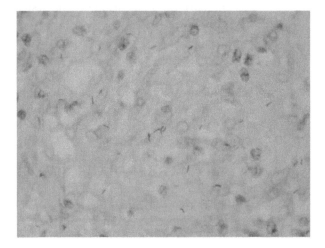

Figure 10.8   Ziehl–Neelsen staining of mycobacteria from a sputum sample

The responsible mycobacteria may be detectable by Ziehl–Neelsen staining (Figure 10.8).

Diagnosis

The diagnosis of TB is suggested by the history and confirmed by:

- Clinical examination
- Massively raised erythrocyte sedimentation rate (ESR)
- Tuberculin skin testing (Mantoux or Heaf test)
- Chest radiography: may show scarring and hilar lymphadenopathy
- Computed tomography (CT): may show areas of calcification or highlight a tuberculous abscess in disseminated disease
- Sputum samples (searching for acid-fast bacilli), see Figure 10.8

- Blood cultures: polymerase chain reaction (PCR) techniques and interferon release assays have accelerated the diagnosis and speciation of mycobacteria
- Bronchoscopy and bronchial washings.

Management

Tuberculosis is a notifiable disease (public health authorities [the Proper Officer of the local authority] must be informed of the diagnosis) and contact tracing is an important aspect of management – with the primary aim of limiting spread of the disease. Antibiotic chemotherapy should be instituted as early as possible and includes:

- For 'asymptomatic' patients: isoniazid for 6 months, or isoniazid and rifampicin for 3 months
- For 'symptomatic sputum-positive' patients: combination chemotherapy of isoniazid, rifampicin and either pyrazimamide or ethambutol for 2 months with continuation of daily isoniazid and rifampicin for a further 4 months
- For HIV-positive individuals with MDR TB: capreomycin has been used effectively.

All anti-tuberculous drugs have potential serious side effects and require careful monitoring. If patient compliance is in question, directly observed therapy (DOT), where drugs are dispensed by and taken in the presence of a health care professional, may be indicated.

Prevention of TB by BCG vaccination (uses live attenuated *Mycobacterium bovis*) is advocated for high-risk individuals and health care professionals, although its efficacy has been questioned.

Oral health care relevance

- Cervical lymphadenopathy is a common feature of TB.
- Oral manifestations are uncommon, but include tuberculous oral nodules or ulceration: the lesions, often on the tongue, having typically undermined margins.
- Anti-tuberculous medication may cause a number of drug interactions with drugs commonly used in dentistry, e.g. rifampicin interacting with azoles and benzodiazepines.
- Oral side effects of anti-tuberculous medication are uncommon, but may include lichenoid lesions due to streptomycin (now only used in severe or multi-drug resistant disease). Additionally, rifampicin can produce an orange-red discolouration of urine and body secretions including the saliva.
- Patients with open TB are likely to be infectious and dental treatment is therefore best delayed until the patient is being treated. If it is not possible to defer treatment then the patient must be treated in a highly controlled environment where the release of infective material into the environment can be minimised and appropriately scavenged.

Syphilis

Syphilis is a sexually transmitted bacterial infection, caused by *Treponema pallidum*, that may damage the cardiovascular or nervous systems or the foetus and potentially can be fatal. Over 80% of cases are in men who have sex with men.

Clinical features

- The incidence of syphilis is rising and, in HIV infection, it can cause a particularly atypical severe form of the disease (lues maligna).
- Primary infection features as a chancre (primary or Hunterian chancre): a painless round indurated ulcer. This often appears within 3 weeks of initial exposure, although it may occur long after. The chancre usually heals spontaneously within 2–3 weeks (the patient, however, remains infected and progresses to secondary syphilis).
- Secondary syphilis features are often non-specific with fever, headache, malaise, a rash (characteristically, symmetrical coppery maculopapules on the palms) and generalised painless lymph node enlargement. These typically present approximately 1–2 months after the appearance of the chancre. Untreated, this will progress to tertiary syphilis.
- Tertiary syphilis can cause cardiovascular lesions (aortitis, coronary arterial stenosis or aortic aneurysms), neurosyphilis or gummas (localised non-infectious granulomas that form deep punched-out ulcers). This stage of the disease may present many years after initial infection.

Clinical signs

Secondary syphilis often manifests with lymphadenopathy and a rash (Figure 10.9) due to the systemic spread of the bacteria. The rash varies in appearance,

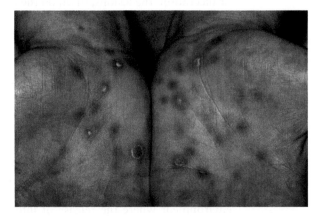

Figure 10.9   Rash due to the systemic spread of the bacteria in secondary syphilis

yet frequently involves the palms and soles. During secondary syphilis, additional symptoms such as fever, general malaise, loss of appetite, muscle aches, joint pain and hair loss may occur. Mucous patches may be seen in or on the mouth, vagina or penis. Moist, warty areas, called condylomata lata, may develop on the genitalia or skin folds, or in the mouth.

Diagnosis

- Diagnosis is by dark-ground microscopy of lesional exudate, and serology.
- Non-specific (reaginic) tests e.g. VDRL (Venereal Disease Research Laboratory), rapid plasma reagin (RPR) card test, automated reagin test (ART) and toluidine red treated serum test (TRUST) are useful for initial screening.
- Specific tests e.g. the fluorescent treponemal antibody (absorbed) (FTA-Abs) test, the *Treponema pallidum* haemagglutination (TPHA) test and the *Treponema pallidum* immobilisation (TPI) test are then needed.

Management

- Syphilis is treated with procaine benzylpenicillin or doxycycline or erythromycin.
- Patients must be followed up clinically and serologically.
- Contacts should be traced.
- Syphilis is a notifiable disease and must be reported in order that potentially infected sexual partners may be identified and treated.

Oral health care relevance

- Syphilitic ulceration should be considered in the differential diagnosis of atypical oral ulceration, particularly as this condition is becoming increasingly common.
  - Primary chancres occasionally involve the lips or tongue.
  - Secondary syphilis can cause highly infectious mouth ulcers (mucous patches and snailtrack ulcers) or condylomas.
  - Tertiary syphilis may manifest intra-orally as a gumma, which may ulcerate or perforate bone, particularly the palate. Additionally leukoplakia, especially of the dorsum of the tongue, may occur at a late stage in the course of the disease and has a high malignant potential.
- Congenital syphilis is a rare cause of learning disability, deafness and blindness (Hutchinson triad) and typically results in frontal bossing (Parrot nodes), a saddle nose, circumoral scarring (rhagades), Hutchinson teeth – screw-driver shaped incisors – and Moon molars.

Index

Printed and bound by CPI Group (UK) Ltd, Croydon, CR0 4YY

27/10/2024

14580389-0001